MW01617023

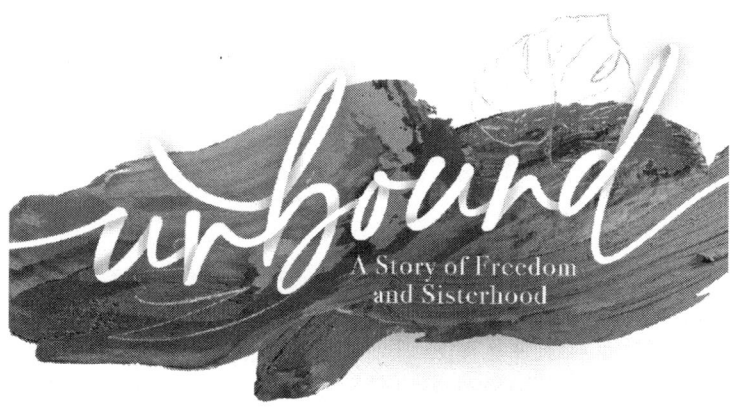

A Story of Freedom
and Sisterhood

TICCOA
LEISTER

Copyright © 2020 Ticcoa Leister

All rights reserved.

ISBN: 978-0-578-76318-7

Cover design by Nicole Grimes

Front cover photo by Stephanie Dove Blake

Front cover stock from
https://creativemarket.com/Lyuart/3050993
-Painted-collection.-Strokescards and
https://creativemarket.com/Lisima/394339
0-Abstract-collection-watercolor-art

To my best sister, Jess —
You taught me how to be brave.
Ohana.

And to #the4500 —
The best group of internet friends.
#the45004LYFE.

Contents

Foreword

Within a few pages, you'll read about the incredible way in which Ticcoa and I met, and watch the friendship between us unfold.

It feels almost cliché to invoke the parable Jesus told of the Good Samaritan here, but I'm doing it anyway. (Hard-roll your eyes, if you must, Ticcoa.)

As readers, you will meet Ticcoa within these pages, and her role as the person found by the Good Samaritan in the biblical story is clear.

Robbed. Beaten. Left for dead on the side of the road. That's how you'll find Ticcoa, too.

Sidestepped by the religious people who should have been the first to come to her aid, there was no other role for me. No, I wasn't the despised Samaritan — that's Someone else, the One in another parable who left the ninety-nine sheep to go after the one who was lost.

You see, when Ticcoa first began exploring the idea of coming to Texas, I was on the verge of becoming an empty-nester. I had several empty bedrooms upstairs because four of my five children had already found their wings. It was a no-brainer to offer her a room, at no charge, while she got on her feet here. Because she had a college degree, an apartment, and a car in South Carolina, I figured she'd land on her feet in no time, here, as well.

I'll leave the rest of the story for Ticcoa to tell, but you should know my role in her story all along was that of the innkeeper: charged by the Good One with taking care of the wounded until their return when the account would be settled between the two of them. As such, I had a front row seat in this unfolding drama.

As I turned the last page of this manuscript, I found myself remembering my own sister, Lillian, whose life and essence was lost too soon, in a whole new way. She has been my sister all along, of course, but because of our age difference and the circumstances when she took me in and finished raising me, I had only ever seen her in that role. She had been the innkeeper in my story as well. And Lillian needed my help, in different ways, just as I needed Ticcoa's: the practical kind ("Hand me your laptop"), as well as the deeper, heart kind. Reading this book helped me remember and further grieve those I loved, bringing more healing to my heart from the trauma of losing them.

As you turn the last page, you'll understand how Ticcoa's life and mine have been so marked by one another's presence, and why I now count her among the "ride or die" sisters my heart chose.

Ticcoa Leister

Anna LeBaron

Author of *The Polygamist's Daughter: A Memoir*

unbound

a story of freedom & sisterhood

Prologue

Adrenaline pulsed through my veins as I clicked the red, telephone-shaped symbol on the screen to end the video call. The last twenty minutes had easily been among the most nerve-wracking moments of my life. The conversation, though silent, was the next step toward the fulfillment of a dream that had been lodged deep in my heart: I was going to Gallaudet University.

My earliest exposure to American Sign Language (ASL) that I remember occurred when I was about eight years old and saw a Deaf couple in line at the grocery store. Their hands moved rapidly as they communicated to one another; my eyes widened as I realized they were having a silent conversation. Fascinated by the fluid movements of their hands and the animated expressions on their faces, a feeling rose deep inside me: one I couldn't articulate or understand at the time. A short time later, my grandparents began attending a large church in a nearby city. When my family visited, my eyes focused on the ASL interpreter the church had positioned at the front of the sanctuary, her hands weaving through the air as she translated the service. Again, I was transfixed. I have been enamored with ASL ever since.

In one week, on July 12, 2013, I would pack my bags, pick up a rental car, and embark on a solo trip to participate in a two-week American Sign Language immersion course in Washington, D.C. Gathering the courage to make this leap had taken years.

Twelve years earlier, when I was seventeen, I sat in the closing worship session of a national drama conference and watched Tyra Lokey, a worship arts teacher who ministered through interpretive movement, dance, and American Sign Language. My best friends and I had attended as many of her workshops as possible throughout the conference. We spent our free periods hanging out at her vendor table, chatting with her, and learning all we could about her ministry to the Deaf community.

During the closing session, I sat in the wing of the balcony, mesmerized by the beauty of the way Tyra worshipped through American Sign Language. It resonated deep in my spirit with something that gave me hope of connecting my fascination with ASL to the world at large; it felt both foreign and familiar. That night, I heard the Holy Spirit speak to my soul, *You could do that.* As this notion soaked into my heart, I responded silently, yet firmly: *I could do that.* Tyra's hands flew through the empty space around her, her hands catching the air and turning it into silent words as I breathed a prayer, "Is this what I'm supposed to do?" While I didn't hear an audible voice respond to my question, I felt a deeply-rooted peace that I had found my calling. I was not quite sure how it would unfold, but I knew ASL and the Deaf community fit somewhere in the equation.

After this experience in 2001, I wrestled with how to integrate my passion for ASL with a future career or ministry. As a very introverted, sheltered young adult, I didn't have a clear vision of the path I wanted to pursue. Upon graduating high school the next year, attending college did not seem like a viable option. Instead I began a full-time job at a local daycare while trying to figure out the answer to the question every new graduate encounters: *What should I do with my life?* I didn't really know what I wanted to do long-term. I was interested in teaching, but far too timid for that profession. ASL interpreting was a consideration, but I didn't know ASL outside the few dozen signs I had learned on the church drama team and, for that matter, I didn't even know anyone who was Deaf. Both these possibilities seemed too far out of reach. I was too shy, too quiet, and too afraid to pursue them.

By the summer of 2005, I had decided to attend North Greenville University, a small, local Christian college. Because I loved children and had no other clear path, I began my college career as an early childhood education major. Before the end of my second semester, I realized that the education program was not for me. I switched my major to English and began cultivating strong relationships with the professors in the English department. Reading and writing had always been my favorite pastimes, and each upper-level English class I took fed those interests; reading novels and literary theory textbooks and writing essays and research papers were almost too fun to be considered work. The only thing missing was the opportunity to study ASL.

I had amassed a collection of ASL dictionaries over the past few years. I taught myself as many signs as I could, using praise and worship music (the slow tempo and repetitive nature of the genre were helpful practice tools) to reinforce what I was learning. Ultimately, though, I wanted formal training: an opportunity to immerse myself in the language and increase my fluency. I felt very strongly that the lack of ASL classes at NGU needed to be addressed, but the possibility of affecting change in this area seemed out of reach until I woke up early one morning my sophomore year with an outline of a plan to propose an ASL course to the curriculum committee. Excitedly, I scribbled notes before getting ready for class.

Later that afternoon, I popped into my advisor's office. Dr. Drummond knew of my interest in ASL and my disappointment that further study was not an option at NGU. As I shared my plan with her, she enthusiastically agreed that we needed to find a way to implement it. She pulled the university handbook out of her desk drawer to see if there was an existing course that would allow me to write a proposal for adding an ASL course while earning credits toward my degree. The next thing I knew, she was leading me across the hall into the English Department Chair's office. Dr. Drummond and I explained my idea to Dr. Collier and asked her advice on how to proceed. She told us to make an appointment with Dr. Sepko, the Dean of Humanities, to obtain approval for me to undertake an independent research writing class under Dr. Drummond's supervision.

When we met with Dr. Sepko, she shared a scripture from Habakkuk to encourage me as I pursued this endeavor: "And the Lord answered me: 'Write the vision; make it plain on tablets so he may run who reads it'" (Habakkuk 2:2, NIV).[1] I had searched for a way to study ASL and Deaf culture while at a university that didn't offer any classes on those topics; I had been given an opportunity to do just that. Days before the spring semester ended, Dr. Sepko approved an independent study that involved writing a research thesis to explain why NGU needed an ASL program, to analyze the availability of and need for ASL programs within a five-state radius, and to define the validity of ASL as a language. I would also complete a survey of both the student body and faculty of NGU to assess the interest level in ASL classes. Throughout the summer, I researched, read, and built my case. During the following semester, I wrote a research thesis and conducted a campus-wide survey, which indicated an overwhelming interest in ASL classes among both students and faculty.

On January 23, 2008 – two years later – I presented an overview of Deaf culture and the history of ASL, a summary of my thesis, and a proposal for the addition of an ASL course at NGU to a faculty panel. At that point, I handed over the proposal to Dr. Sepko, as well as the head of the Curriculum Committee, and the chair of the Foreign Language department. The events that were orchestrated and the key people who I encountered during this process convinced me that the idea I awoke to that April morning had been divinely appointed.

As with any institutional process, the wait between the time I submitted my proposal to the curriculum committee and the first ASL class on campus was a long one. So long, in fact, that I graduated before the fruit of my labor came to life. But in January 2011, one year after

I graduated from NGU, I sat in the front row during the very first ASL class on NGU's campus, completely in awe as I watched the vision God had placed in my heart unfold before my eyes. When the class ended, I approached the instructor, Shannon Fike and extended my hand. "Hi, I'm Ticcoa. I've been praying for you for years. I'm so glad you're finally here."

While writing my thesis, I used 1 Corinthians 3:6-7 as a foundational scripture for my work: "I planted, Apollos watered, but God gave the growth. So, neither he who plants nor he who waters is anything, but only God who gives the growth" (ESV).[2] I had planted the seed with my proposal and presentation; the curriculum committee and the professors who supported the proposal kept it moving forward; and God ultimately grew the program into what it is today. A decade after I wrote my proposal, NGU now offers sixteen ASL and Deaf culture classes, an ASL minor and Interdisciplinary Studies component, and employs four ASL instructors.

As influential as the proposal I wrote was, it took me a long time to own my role in the process of finally bringing ASL to NGU. In fact, until a conversation I had with a counselor in 2016, I believed that anybody could have done this. But God hadn't asked just anybody to do this crazy thing. He'd asked me, and had equipped me to do exactly what he called me to do. God planted the seed of a burning zeal for ASL and the Deaf community in my heart and coaxed it to life. This process and experience fanned the flame of my passion for ASL and the Deaf community even more, motivating me to begin exploring options for a master's degree in teaching ASL, which is how I found myself headed to Gallaudet to stick my toes in the water of ASL and Deaf culture immersion.

I audited ASL I, II, and III at my alma mater, building my vocabulary and becoming more comfortable with facial grammar and the structural components of ASL. As you might imagine, a master's degree in ASL is not an easy degree to come by. Acceptance of ASL as a valid, stand-alone language is still not widespread. Many misconceptions exist about ASL and the Deaf community. There are a handful of related programs across the country, but the most well-respected one is Gallaudet University's M.A.T. in Sign Language.

Gallaudet University (affectionately known as "Gally" by the Deaf community) is the only university whose programs are specifically designed for students who are deaf or hard-of-hearing, thereby making it a truly immersive environment for Deaf culture. It is considered the core of education in the Deaf community, and it became my goal to study there.

But I was so scared to act on it. Entering any new culture and learning any new, non-native language is uncomfortable; for my sheltered, introverted heart, it was terrifying. Many soul-searching conversations with my friends, mentors, and former professors took place before I was remotely ready to move toward attending Gallaudet. In the spring of 2013, I felt that it was time. I pored over the graduate school website, requested application materials, and decided to visit the program over the summer. I also enrolled in a two-week ASL immersion course to gauge the pace and atmosphere of classes at Gallaudet, which was to take place in July.

Chapter 1:

Robbed

As the service closed, Pastor C invited members who wanted prayer to come to the front of the dimly-lit church. Anxious about being the center of attention, I silently wrestled with whether I should go to the front of the room. I'd just received my application and information packet from the graduate school at Gallaudet University in the mail that week, and was both excited and overwhelmed by the possibilities it brought.

That Sunday morning in April 2013, as I stood in the row of chairs on the far side of the sanctuary, a male church member approached me.

"Do you want prayer?" he asked.

I shrugged, noncommittally.

"You should go," he urged.

I supposed I should. After all, wasn't this the best place to obtain God's stamp of approval on my plans? Wasn't the pastor's wisdom valuable in my decision-making? Everything I had been taught about faith and God's will said *yes*. I slid out of the row of blue fabric chairs, and slowly walked to the small group of people lined up in the aisle in front of the pastor. My heart was beating hard and fast.

When my turn came, a small circle of church members was gathered around the pastor. I approached him.

"I'm going to Gallaudet this summer to take an immersion class and visit the graduate school. I need prayer for provision, wisdom, and direction about taking this step."

He held out his hands, beckoning me to place mine in his. I did. The circle of people enclosed us and other members placed their hands on my back, shoulders, and arms. We closed our eyes and he prayed for exactly what I had asked. When he finished, I thanked him and returned to my seat.

After the service, my family was among the last to leave. A few other people milled around the sanctuary, chatting with one another. Pastor C was sitting on the front row of chairs, watching a few of the children, including my niece, play with one another in front of the platform. I walked by them and he asked me to sit.

"Thanks for the prayer," I said as I sat down.

He had not looked at me yet, his eyes still on the children.

"This is not what you're supposed to do. If you go down this path, you will get hurt," he instructed, matter-of-factly.

His words cut through my mind like a knife. My brain scrambled to comprehend what he was saying. My breath caught in my chest, and my stomach dropped. He turned, looking at me now with imploring eyes.

"I love you like a father, and I don't want to hurt you, but if you pursue this you will get hurt," he reiterated.

Unable to speak, I managed a weak nod and sober half-smile. My heart was crushed. Shattered. Grieving. I managed to keep my face from crumbling until I exited the building. I told my mom and sister that I would not be home for lunch and climbed into my car. Stunned and in shock, I drove aimlessly for hours in silence. I was numb.

Later that evening, when I finally went home, I was exhausted from the emotional trauma, though I did not know what it was at the time. I got in the shower and let the hot water rain over me as if it would wash away the pain I was in. The tears that I had held back all day began to flow. Deep, gut-wrenching sobs poured out of my body as I huddled in the corner of the shower, my face buried in a towel so my family would not hear me upstairs. It felt as though something in me had been ripped away.

Half an hour later, I emerged from the shower, depleted. I crawled into bed where I tossed and turned all night, getting very little sleep. My total excitement had turned into a nightmare.

The next morning, the deep soreness of my abdominal muscles added to the ache of my heart. I stumbled through the motions of getting dressed and driving to the school where I worked as an assistant teacher.

My co-teacher, Christine, and I had been close since I first walked into her classroom as a behavioral therapy aide for one of her students three years earlier in the fall of 2010. When I met her, I instantly felt a connection with her and we formed a fast friendship. By the end of the semester, her assistant teacher had decided she would not be returning the next year. Christine asked me if I would be interested in taking her place, and I said yes without hesitation. We had worked together for five-and-a-half years and by this point were a dynamic duo, well-loved by both our students and their parents. Not only did we spend our weekdays together, but we also spent lots of time at the library or coffee shops, each of us completing assignments for the degrees we were pursuing.

While I was usually the first one to arrive in our classroom, Christine had beaten me there that morning. As I opened the classroom door and entered, her back was to me as she prepared the room.

"Good morning," she said as she began to run down our plans for the day.

Before I had a chance to return the greeting, Christine turned around to face me. As soon as she looked at me, she knew something was wrong. She stopped, mid-sentence, concern etched on her face. My countenance must have clearly indicated how devastated I was.

"Are you okay?" she gently asked. "What happened?"

Again, my mask began to crumble as I shook my head, willing the torrent of tears not to burst forth. Our classroom would soon fill with kindergartners and I wasn't sure I would be able to rein in my emotions before they arrived. My voice cracked as I gave her a brief synopsis of the previous day's events.

"Pastor C told me not to go to Gallaudet. He said I would be hurt if I go," I whispered. "No explanation, that's it. I'll get hurt and this is not what I'm supposed to do."

Christine's eyebrows drew together in suspicion. She knew how excited I was about attending Gallaudet that summer and was shocked at Pastor C's declaration.

Knowing he had recently had heart surgery, she grasped for an explanation.

"I've heard that people just aren't the same after such major surgery," she mused. "Maybe this has something to do with that."

I shrugged, too weary to try to find an answer. Knowing our students would begin arriving within minutes, I excused myself to put away my belongings. Then, I ducked into the restroom to pull myself together. Even though I felt like the earth had given way beneath me, I put my mask back on and pretended I was okay.

It was no secret to anyone who knew me that the Deaf community and American Sign Language held a special place in my heart. Several times, I had requested to sign songs as it was my favorite way to express praise and worship. Pastor C had encouraged me to do so, which made his declaration very hard for me to understand.

We did not have a close personal relationship. In fact, our conversations had been few and brief in the five years I had attended the church. Still, I had grown up in a Deep South, evangelical church culture that placed a high value on respecting and obeying the authority of church leadership. And my people-pleasing tendencies that were developed when I was a young child meant I was easily convinced to heed the warnings of authority figures.

For a few weeks after seeking prayer, I struggled with knowing whether Pastor C's words were true. Had I heard the Holy Spirit wrong? Were all the events of the last few years a tease? Was this love for ASL and the Deaf community ingrained in me for nothing? Those closest to me — the people who had been alongside me as I explored this passion — all counseled me that I was supposed to pursue this path; they believed it was what I was supposed to do as much as I did. When I relayed what Pastor C had said, they were as dumbfounded by it as Christine had been.

I prayed, begging God to give me clear direction, but my confidence in my ability to hear had been skewed. I was poised to follow what I understood as God's calling to immersion learning and graduate school at Gallaudet. I was ready. I was willing. I was determined. I had prayed about it. I had researched it. I had applied for it. I had interviewed for it. I had enrolled. I was excited about it. And then one conversation, in a seemingly safe place, brought it all crashing down.

Ultimately, I decided that I would follow through with my plans to visit Gallaudet and take the immersion class. A week before the trip, on July 4, I completed a video interview and assessment with the ASL department chair at Gallaudet to make sure my skill level was appropriate for the course I'd chosen. Despite the blurry internet connection and several technical difficulties, I completed the assessment and received validation of my signing skills from the instructor. All that was left to do was pack for my trip and pick up my rental car on July 12, the night before I left for Gallaudet.

"You're all set." The employee at the rental car agency handed me the key to a burgundy Dodge Charger.

"Great, thanks," I said as I took the keys and paperwork from him.

Dashing out the door and through a light summer rain, I climbed into the driver's seat. My sister, Jess, got in beside me. I started the car and pulled onto the highway. Within minutes it began to rain harder. Soon, it was pouring so hard I could barely see the road. I decided to stop on the side of the road and wait until it cleared.

Jess and I chatted and tried to figure out how to operate the radio and air conditioner while we waited. Finally, the rain let up enough to continue the drive home.

Shifting the gear stick into drive, I pressed the accelerator. The car didn't move. I tried again. Nothing. Again. The car did not move. Dread rising, I told Jess to find the car manual to troubleshoot. While she flipped through the pages, my thoughts raced.

This is what he meant. You can't even drive a car. If you go, you will get hurt. You might have a wreck. You might get mugged. You might get lost. You might have a heart attack. You might get raped. What if you have car trouble? What if you fail? What if he's right? What if you get hurt? What if this is not what you're supposed to do? How do you know you heard God? He's the pastor: who are you to question his discernment? What if...What if...What if....

The worst-case scenarios taunted me. Doubt flooded me. Anxiety overtook me. My breathing became low and shallow. I felt like there was a cement block sitting on my chest.

In the midst of this, Jess realized that that car was a semi-automatic and I had been trying to put it in drive while in manual mode. I managed to calm down enough to put the car in the correct gear and start toward home again. But by now, my thoughts had gone off the cliff of reason. My brain was overwhelmed. Although I didn't recognize it as such then, I was experiencing my first full-blown panic attack.

For the twenty-minute drive to the house, I thought of everything that could possibly go wrong with this trip. No longer confident that I was making the right choice, I could not get Pastor C's words out of my head.

The fear that I was making a huge mistake paralyzed me.

We arrived home, where I had planned to load my suitcases into the car so I would be ready for my early departure the next morning. Instead, I headed to my basement apartment, wrestling with my thoughts.

If you go, you will get hurt.

Drained, I stopped packing my bags and went to bed. The next morning, after a sleepless night, I texted my friend, Kate, who I was supposed to stay with in a suburb outside of D.C.

"Just wanted to let you know that I've canceled my trip, so you won't see me tonight."

I returned the rental car that afternoon, robbed of my confidence to make wise decisions, my peace, and the ability to envision a future of possibility.

Chapter 2:

Flatlined

Silvery threads of light cut through the gap in the blackout curtains that shrouded the window above my bed. Huddled under a fluffy comforter to ward off the chill of an unseasonably cold October night, I burrowed myself into bed. My heart was heavy after yet another argument with Mom. Discouraged that I couldn't mold myself to her standards and shake myself loose from the grip depression had on me, I felt hope slipping away. I wasn't the perfect eldest daughter setting a good example for my siblings; I was barely slogging through each day. I showed up in my classroom with a happy face pasted on for my students because I believed they were worth showing up for, but my eyes were empty. Whatever scrap of belief I'd found in myself when I decided to pursue Gallaudet had shriveled. At twenty-nine years old, my dreams were dead. I didn't have the strength or the blessing or the favor to go after what lit up my soul. And if I wasn't supposed to do the one thing that made me come alive with passionate vigor, what was the point in even being alive, merely surviving day after day after day? Was it really God's plan for me to just go through the motions every day so I wouldn't get hurt? I pulled the blanket over my head, tears rolling down my cheeks.

If this is how it's going to be, I don't want to wake up tomorrow, I prayed.

If I said I opened my eyes the next morning, joyfully alive, it would be a lie. Instead, I awoke resigned to merely surviving in the wake of my shattered dreams. Emotionally, I was flatlining. Dead.

The decision not to go to Gallaudet that summer because of someone else's opinion of my calling damaged my heart and mind in ways I never imagined it would. I spent the largest part of the next two years in a dark hole. All those relentless tormentors — Fear, Anxiety, Depression, Lies, Regret, Numbness — they all took their turns beating their way into my mind and soul. And once they arrived, they weren't going anywhere anytime soon. They moved in and made themselves at home.

Before Pastor C's declaration, I was excited about what the future held. I felt God speaking into the very depths of my soul about what I should be pursuing. He'd already pulled me out of my comfort zone and led me down a trail I'd never expected to be walking.

Then, my dreams crashed around me. I shut down; I became a shell of myself. I lost my joy, my motivation, my belief that God could speak to me. Though I put on a mask of "everything's okay" every day, and went through the motions of my life, those closest to me knew I was struggling.

I struggled to stay afloat, to care, to believe in God's goodness, to believe I was enough in every area: as a daughter, a sister, a friend, a teacher, etc. My self-worth plummeted. If I could have stayed in bed twenty-four hours of every day for the remainder of 2013 and most of 2014, I would have. I was depressed, ashamed, and broken.

What I didn't know then was that depression and anxiety manifest themselves in a variety of ways. It doesn't just look like staying in bed and crying all day. It looks like letting regular household chores slide, like papers piling up on every available surface, like floors covered with laundry piles that may or may not be clean. It looks like canceling plans with friends at the last minute. It looks like shutting down and isolating yourself from the people closest to you. It looks like not having physical, mental, or emotional energy to deal with any sort of conflict. It looks like doing the bare minimum to survive.

Because I was living in the half-finished basement apartment at my mom's house, this created a strain on our relationship. As the oldest of four siblings, I felt tremendous pressure to be the perfect example. And I was failing miserably. While I never actually had a plan to end my life, I often thought that it would be better if I weren't alive anymore because I would no longer be such a disappointment to everyone who knew me.

Pastor C's opinion had plunged me headfirst into a deep pit of shame, fear, regret, numbness, feeling like I would never see the light of day again. And because our family dynamic was chronically dysfunctional, I never learned how to process, deal with, or express my emotions in healthy ways. It was the darkest season I had ever known. I had shown up in the arena and had been pummeled to the ground.

The aftermath of hearing Pastor C declare my calling invalid robbed me of my life. I distanced myself from those closest to me because I feared disappointing them, especially four of my former college professors who had become my friends. They were the ones who supported me and cheered me on during the process of bringing ASL to North Greenville University, who had encouraged me to pursue Gallaudet. But I was afraid and embarrassed for them to know that I had canceled my trip.

I poured all of my energy into showing up in my classroom every weekday morning. The smiles and laughter from my students kept me from sinking completely into the darkness that lurked around the edges of my life. I will always be grateful for the solace that my co-teacher, our students, and our classroom offered that year. I still felt like I had a purpose, if not the one I felt was my true calling.

But as much comfort and distraction as being in the classroom brought, it was only a bandage applied to the bleeding wounds that had been inflicted on my soul.

Chapter 3:

#the4500

"You are my people."
Jen Hatmaker

The silence of the library was thick as I scrolled through Facebook. Since moving into an apartment with a friend from college a few months earlier, I had developed the habit of spending a couple of hours after work at the library across the street. I paused at a post from a popular blogger I was following, clicked over to her blog, and read about her new book that would be released in the fall. She was extending an invitation for her readers to be on the launch team: an opportunity to read the book in advance of its release. I had never heard of a launch team, but was intrigued.

For the next few days, the launch team frequently came to mind, but I was sure I wouldn't make the team if I applied. After all, I had very few social media followers and knew that numbers mattered to publishers when it came to opportunities such as this one. Heck, I had not even posted anything on my blog for more than a year. There was no way I would get picked for the team.

But I couldn't stop thinking about it. After Gallaudet slipped from my grasp and depression had taken over my life, I stopped reading and writing for pleasure. Both activities required more mental bandwidth and emotional energy than I had. The emotion was too raw, the rejection too near, and the questions too unresolved. But I began to feel the bubble of the unwritten words that filled my heart. The burden of an untold story is heavy, especially for a writer. Too many thoughts in my head at once are overwhelming when writing has always been my processing outlet.

So, the fact that this launch team even remotely interested me was unusual. If nothing else, it would be a way to get back into the habit of reading and writing while helping support a blogger whose writing I already enjoyed. A few days later, I was sitting in the library after work again. I typed in the author's blog name and made my way back to the post about the launch team, filled out the application, and clicked submit.

"*Thank you for applying to Jen Hatmaker's For the Love Launch Team....*"The confirmation message flashed as I stared at the computer screen. The date was March 7, 2015. The last day the application was open. I'd slid in just hours before the deadline.

Three days later — Friday, March 10, 2015 — an email arrived in my inbox. Subject line: *Thanks for Applying to the For the Love Launch Team!* I opened the email to find that I had, unfortunately, not been selected for the launch team. I kept reading. The publisher included four chapters of the books as a consolation prize of sorts for those of us who were not on the launch team. The email also included a note from Jen. In her enthusiastic, gushing way, she explained that she would have wanted us all and declared, "YOU ARE MY PEOPLE!"

Disappointed but not surprised that I was one of the 4,500 people — out of 5,000 applicants — who had not been selected for the launch team, I was still happy to have the four chapters of Jen's new book to read. I tore through them quickly the next day, laughing and crying as her words resonated deep inside me.

The following Monday, Jen's social media accounts became a gathering place for both the launch team and those who hadn't been chosen. On her Facebook page, Jen posted about the overwhelming response her invitation had brought. There were thousands of comments that declared some variation of either "I'm on the team!" or "I didn't make it," accompanied by emojis of celebration and despair, respectively. I added my own disappointment to the cacophony of virtual voices on Jen's post. Her post also talked about how someone had tweeted her and used a hashtag, #the4500, that was now trending on her Twitter feed. I opened Twitter and went to Jen's feed to see what was happening for myself but didn't reply to any of the tweets.

Later that day, I got a notification that someone had replied to my comment on Jen's Facebook post. I clicked the notification to read the comment from someone named Anna: "If you didn't get an email, or didn't even apply, you can join our FB group (search #the4500). We will band together to promote #ForTheLove. ALL ARE WELCOME TO JOIN THE PARTY!!!"

What have I stumbled upon, here? I wondered. At that point, I had a very surface-level relationship with social media. I had grown up in the first generation of social media users--the ones who had been urgently warned against interaction with strangers on the internet. I wasn't Facebook friends with anyone I had never met in person and even then I was judicious about who I allowed into my private cyber life. But now I had something in common with all of these internet strangers.

Still, I was wary of joining a Facebook group filled with hundreds of people I didn't know in real life. If my memory is accurate, it was about a week before my curiosity won and I requested to join the Facebook group, #the4500.

Once I was in the group, my news feed was bombarded with posts and notifications from the group. It was a nonstop, twenty-four-hour party. Approximately 1300 of the 4500 launch team rejects had joined and were getting to know one another. The introduction posts quickly gave way to deeper stories as tight-knit friendships were born. But just as I was an introverted wallflower in real life, I lurked in the corners of #the4500's virtual room. The flood of notifications was overwhelming, so I turned them off and only caught what was in my newsfeed. I liked a post here and there, but mostly went on with my regular life.

My first post in the group was in April 2015: a short, sweet anecdote about something that had happened in my classroom that day. I never made an introduction post. My comments never revealed anything deeper than surface-level information. My first friend request from a group member came that month, too. It was from Anna, one of the group administrators. I let that request sit in my notifications for quite a while before I accepted it, nervous about letting someone I did not actually know into my online life.

At that point, I only knew a few things about Anna. 1) She had originally tweeted Jen and used #the4500 when the launch team rejection email went out. 2) She was a co-admin of the Facebook group with another woman, Tracy. Tracy had swooped up Anna's hashtag from Twitter and used it as the name of her Facebook group. Then, the two of them connected on Jen's Facebook post and became fast friends and co-admins of the group. 3) Anna liked and commented on ALL the posts in the Facebook group. That she was a ball of boundless energy and enthusiasm was clear even through cyberspace. But she seemed safe enough to be friends with on Facebook, so I accepted her request.

For the next few months, I continued lurking in the group, posting about little moments of my life a handful of times, still not revealing anything deeply personal. Sometime during the summer, Anna followed me on Twitter, and I followed her back. But her bio caught my eye: "I'm writing a book about escaping my father's violent, polygamist cult." *Um, what? Polygamist cult? Who is this woman?* She seemed normal enough in the Facebook group, but this new information definitely gave me pause. *Okay, lady. We can be Facebook friends, but you stay over there in your corner of the internet and I'll stay over here in mine.*

One Sunday near the end of July, I was at my mom's house for lunch with my family. After we ate, I was sitting in the living room, scrolling through the group when a brightly-colored quote graphic caught my eye. It was a Theodore Roosevelt quote from Brené Brown's book, *Daring Greatly: How the Courage to Be Vulnerable Transforms the Way We Live, Love, Parent, and Lead*[1]:

"It is not the critic who counts; not the man who points out how the strong man stumbles, or where the doer of deeds could have done them better. The credit belongs to the man who is actually in the arena, whose face is marred by dust and sweat and blood; who strives valiantly; [...] who at the best knows in the end the triumph of high achievement, and who at the worst, if he fails, at least fails while daring greatly."

A few posts farther down the feed, I came across another post of Anna's that had been bumped. I slowed my scroll to read the post that Anna had written back in March. Someone had recently commented on it and brought it to the top of the group's feed. Anna's post read, "If you are new to #the4500 and you see me bump some conversation threads back up to the top of the group, I'M DOING THIS FOR YOU!!! I'm also secretly doing it for those of you 'lurkers' that read these conversations quietly without commenting hoping to draw you out. You are part of this group for a reason and your voice matters. If you are afraid to speak out or speak up, that *Daring Greatly* post I keep bumping IS FOR YOU. YES...YOU!!! (You know who you are.)"

She was talking to me. For the first time since I had joined the group, I felt seen. Called out of the shadows. Exposed. I scrolled back to the post about *Daring Greatly*, then opened another browser window and ordered the book. Even though I had seen Anna's post about Brené Brown many times, I finally felt like it was time to read her book.

The book arrived in mid-August and I began reading. Within a few pages, Brown's words brought an aching relief. The ache came from all the raw emotions that had accumulated over the past two years, and even before that growing up in a dysfunctional home. The relief came because I was beginning to understand why the Gallaudet incident and the resulting depression had devastated me so tremendously. The shame of failing and disappointing others had awakened what Brown calls "shame gremlins" that annihilated my self-confidence and sense of worthiness.

According to Brown, "Shame hates having words wrapped around it. If we speak shame, it begins to wither. Just the way exposure to light was deadly for the gremlins, language and story bring light to shame and destroy it." [3] Through her research, she has found that vulnerability, shame, and joy are all closely connected. Because I had been vulnerable when I approached Pastor C and asked for prayer about Gallaudet, then was inundated with shame after his declaration triggered my spiral into depression, I had lost my ability to find joy in almost everything.

For the first time, someone had given me the language to describe everything I'd felt for the last two years. The shame of letting fear talk me out of pursuing my dreams and the debilitating belief that I would never have the gumption to break out of old patterns were holding me hostage. As I read, Brown's words allowed me to come to the realization that I was not crazy for feeling this way and there was hope of living a more authentic life. I knew I needed to begin showing up for my life and reengage with the world around me rather than continuing to just go through the motions and survive each day. But after living in the darkness of depression for years, I was no longer sure how to find the way back to the light, to the real me who was buried deep inside.

Daring Greatly was full of information that I needed to digest slowly. Having mostly read nonfiction books in the explicitly Christian personal development genre (from authors such as Beth Moore, Joyce Meyer, Max Lucado, etc.), reading a self-help book that was not explicitly biblically-based was new territory aside from a few textbooks and research articles in college. Because of how the evangelical worldview permeated my entire life, I found myself suspicious of an author who didn't explicitly reference the Bible or God in her writing. Yet, her

Ticcoa Leister

research and personal experience made sense to my brain
and made me feel less alone in my own life.

And then, I had a dream.

Chapter 4:

The Dream

"...weeping may stay for the night,
but rejoicing comes in the morning."
Psalm 30:5b

My eyes scanned the bustling room. Hundreds of women mingled, filling coffee cups at the coffee bar, embracing one another with wide smiles and gleeful laughter, and scurrying to find seats. I knew no one in the room, and yet I felt like I belonged here with them. My gaze landed upon a woman I recognized from the internet, and made my way toward her.

"Hi, I'm Anna!" she announced as I approached. Her introduction was almost entirely unnecessary. I knew who she was. Everyone was here because of her and Tracy, the co-admins of the Facebook group we were all part of. We chatted for a few moments, and in an uncharacteristically authentic way, I shared how I had been shrouded in a cloak of depression for the last two years. She asked gentle questions and encouraged me that it would not always feel this way, but that I would feel alive again.

"Hey, Anna!" Another woman walked up to greet us, and I felt a little deflated that our conversation was over. As I was about to turn and walk away to avoid an awkward moment, Anna welcomed the newcomer into our circle and continued to speak to me. Her passionate belief that I would find my way out of the pit I was in and be able to live my life in freedom had lightened my heart; I felt a twinge of joy spark deep in my soul.

"Okay girls, let's get started!" Tracy tapped the microphone at the front of the room, calling us to attention.

The shrill beep of the alarm clock interrupted Tracy's voice as my phone vibrated on the nightstand. It was Friday, September 18, 2015. I rolled over and turned off the alarm, but not before realizing that there was a lightness in my heart that had been absent for years.

Instead of hitting the snooze option, I stopped the alarm and noted that waking up this morning was so much different than it had been for the hundreds of nights that had passed since the summer of 2013. Oddly, the urge to pull the blankets over my head and hide from the world wasn't there.

Then I remembered the dream.

I'd met Anna. I'd been in the same room with all the women from #the4500. We'd finally been in the same space in real life, not just in our tight-knit virtual community. As I watched from the wings of the group, I had noticed Anna's bubbly personality among the 1300 women there and particularly the way she invited everyone to pull up a chair and be themselves in the group. She offered encouragement, wisdom, empathy, and compassion that translated even through cyberspace.

The others in the group did not know who I was since I'd posted in the group only a handful of times. I observed from the shadows. Unlike many of these women, I had not connected with anyone on a more personal level. I'd watched photos of in-person meetups come across the pages of the group, but never felt inclined to invest time in getting to know any of them or sharing anything about myself. I was perfectly happy on the fringes.

But when I woke up from the dream that morning, I felt like a weight had rolled off my shoulders. The joy inside me was palpable, yet foreign. None of my circumstances had changed. Posting about the dream in the group crossed my mind, but I thought, *No, that's ridiculous. Nobody will care that you dreamed about this.*

Ten minutes later, I posted, thinking it was just a fun little anecdote that we could all laugh about. I wrote:

"I dreamed of #the4500 last night. The whole legion of us was at some conference and I kept running into people I recognized. We had dinners, coffees, chats together. But what really takes the cake—the moment when I was pouring my heart out to Anna and someone walked up and unintentionally interrupted. Without missing a beat, Anna steered the conversation back to what was on my heart in the gentlest way. I've never met her IRL, but I imagine that she's just as sweet, encouraging, and darling as she was in my dream. Anna—you're a cheerleader for us even in our dreams! It's ridiculous, but I woke up light-hearted and joyful because of our 'dream-chat!'"

Anna was the first to respond.

"We should talk soon!"

Almost immediately, people who had already met her in person were commenting that she really was that sweet in real life. Within ten minutes of posting, I had a private message from Anna, saying, "Here's my number, let's chat!"

Have I mentioned that I'm an introvert? Asking me to talk on the phone is akin to inviting me to a torture session. The thought of an unsolicited call makes me cringe. It's just not an activity I enjoy. Small talk is excruciating. I hate it. But this internet "stranger" wanted to talk to me on the phone. As we say in the South, *bless her extroverted heart.*

Her message needled me all day. When I got home from work, I messaged her back. In total honesty, I told her I was not a fan of phone conversations, but I would love to chat about the book. I asked if we could text instead and gave her my number, so I could not chicken out. Minutes later, my phone buzzed, alerting me to a text. It was Anna. We texted for a few minutes about the book and then she asked where I lived. I told her I was in upstate South Carolina and she replied with a statement that made me believe this was bigger than just having a dream: "My boss just told me today that I'm coming to Charlotte, North Carolina at the end of October! I smell a meetup."

Wait a second, I thought, my mind racing. The very day I wake up from a dream about meeting her, her boss tells her he's flying her from Texas to company headquarters which just happens to be only two hours from me? In a month-and-a-half? Needless to say, I was flabbergasted. Clearly, God was up to something. Nothing else made sense. The circumstances were too perfectly aligned to chalk them up to coincidence. I decided then that I was not going to miss this chance at a meetup. We texted for

a while longer, marveling at what had transpired because
of my dream.

The difference in my mood and attitude during the days
that followed was so markedly changed. I started engaging
with the women in the group, even sending a few of them
friend requests. Over the weekend, I told my sister all
about #the4500, my dream, and the conversation I'd had
with Anna. I felt like I had finally awakened from the fog.

By Tuesday of the following week, a mere five days after
the dream, I was nearly finished reading *Daring Greatly*
and needed to talk it out with someone who had read it.
That evening, I took a leap and texted Anna: "If I was
feeling brave, are you available to talk tonight?" The
introvert was poking her head out of her shell. Anna said
yes, and we agreed on a time.

I was so far outside of my comfort zone. My heart
pounded when my ringtone sounded, the screen showing
a Texas number. I hardly remember what we said that
night, but the time passed so quickly that when I hung up
the phone, I was shocked to see we had chatted for nearly
two hours. Looking back, I recognize that conversation as
a mile marker in the journey I did not yet know I was
taking. I was not aware of how much that one catalytic
moment would change the course of my life in the coming
months. I had been dead inside for too long. Breaking out
of that grave of depression seemed impossible from the
inside. Yet, something in that my dream and the first

conversation with Anna unlocked the recesses of my heart that were holding me fearful and captive, a prisoner of circumstance, choice, perceived failure, wastefulness. It was a tiny ray of light poking into the darkness.

Chapter 5:

Unbound

Meeting Anna in my dream sparked a bit of hope that my life would not always be so deeply saturated with darkness. I came out of the shadows in #the4500 and began commenting, and even posting, more frequently. I accepted a few more friend requests from members of the group, slowly widening the circle of internet friends. As I continued to read *Daring Greatly*, Anna and I texted back-and-forth, which allowed me to further process what I was learning. I later learned that this was a miracle in itself, because Anna strongly dislikes texting long conversations and would much prefer to pick up the phone and chat voice-to-voice. But because I was so opposed to phone calls, she made a rare exception. Occasionally, though, I would feel comfortable with talking on the phone.

During these conversations, Anna provided a listening ear and shared her own experiences with me. She encouraged me to reconnect with God and the Holy Spirit. Anna provided me with a safe, objective space to explore the unhealthy patterns that kept me from living in freedom.

She also introduced me to Bob Hamp, a licensed counselor and biblical teacher in Dallas, TX. I began reading his books and listening to his podcasts in which he offers a perspective of freedom and relationship with God unlike any I had heard before. During this time, I also began writing again. Within a week of my first phone call with Anna, I had revived my blog and began recording the transformation happening in me.

I was processing a lot of experiences and feelings that I had suppressed, numbed, and buried for the past twenty-eight months. This new awareness of my emotional health brought a rather uncomfortable sensation that I was coming out of the shell where I'd been hiding. At one point, I remember describing it to the women in #the4500 as a momentum of bravery that I did not want to lose. For once in a long time, I felt alive again.

And people around me were beginning to notice. Though I had mentioned #the4500 briefly to my mom and sister,

I had not shared a lot of details with them. But the more invested I became in the group, the harder it was to keep my virtual life and real life separated. My family was in awe of how enthusiastic I was when it came to this group of internet strangers. When I visited my former professors on campus one day, my friend Dr. Drummond looked at me seriously and said, "You don't look dead anymore. Your countenance has changed." Her blunt observation did not offend me; I knew the joy that was being reignited inside me was finding its way to the outside of me. I could not contain it. My co-teacher, Christine, noticed the change in my demeanor too. She even asked if I had met a guy when I arrived at work one morning, grinning at something that had happened in the group.

"No, I didn't meet a guy," I replied, laughing, as we reset our classroom for the day. "I met a bunch of women on the internet!" I was head-over-heels in love with #the4500.

The first large group gathering, The Splendid Retreat, was taking place at the end of October in Wisconsin. Tracy and Anna had started planning it in the early days of #the4500, but since I was a lurker and still highly skeptical about what was unfolding in front of me then, I had not even remotely entertained the idea of traveling states away to spend a long weekend with a bunch of internet strangers. Now, as the retreat got closer, I felt a pang of regret that I was not attending the retreat.

One night, after my nightly virtual visit with my friends, I crawled into bed, tired but content. Many of my new friends lived in Texas and, as I drifted off to sleep, I thought, *Maybe I'll go to Texas to visit them someday.* Ironically, Texas had never been on my travel bucket list. I had never had any desire to visit; now, I couldn't wait to go. The problem was that I had never flown at all (nor did I want to fly), or even traveled alone, for that matter. And because I had experienced my worst panic attack in the rental car that was supposed to take me on my solo trip to Gallaudet, going to Texas seemed like a very improbable destination. But, that night, it was nice to think of it as a slight possibility. Someday.

The next morning, September 28, I woke up early for work, rolled over to turn off my alarm, and picked up my phone. As usual, I opened the Facebook app and navigated to #the4500. The first post I saw was Tracy's. She'd written no words: it was just a picture of a field full of bluebonnets. The picture's text overlay jolted me awake in disbelief.

Splendid in the Hills
April 2016
Somewhere in TX

Are you kidding me? I just thought last night that maybe I'd go meet these internet strangers in Texas someday. And I wake up to this post? I was astounded. When Tracy posted the event details and registration link a week later, I was among the first to sign up (in the middle of the night, no less). Though I had no idea how I would work out the logistics, and my anxiety at the thought of traveling alone to Texas was already increasing, I knew I wanted to be there. It felt as though all of these circumstances were being orchestrated in my favor.

Throughout October, November, and December, I spent as much of my free time as possible in #the4500, letting myself be seen in the group but also still doing a lot of observing. More friend requests came and I began sending some of my own, too. In November, Anna met her cousin, Ruth Wariner, on Twitter and ended up launching her book, *The Sound of Gravel*, in November and December. A smaller offshoot group of us from #the4500 banded together under Anna's guidance in Ruth's launch team. The two hundred people in the launch team shared twenty copies of the advance reader copy of *The Sound of Gravel*. We sped through the book then put them in the mail to the next person on the list, including tissues and notes in the packages.

When the book arrived at my mom's house, I went straight there after work to retrieve it, knowing I was on a tight deadline to read it and send it to the next reader. But mom had already opened the package and started reading. I was nervous about what she would think because I had not told her much about Anna's family of origin. (I had spent a lot of time researching it since I began forming a closer friendship with Anna.) She was several chapters in and already hooked. I took the book home with me, and even though it was the middle of the week, I stayed up until 2:00 a.m. reading. Then I woke at 5:00 a.m. to finish before heading to work. I was a total zombie the next day but it was worth it.

That afternoon, I texted Anna and asked if it was okay to keep the book an extra day so Mom could finish reading it. She agreed with the condition that Mom would join the launch team and write a review. So, I put Mom in the launch team group and she finished reading Ruth's story. She was also able to interact with and get to know Anna better.

As the end of 2015 neared, several women in #the4500 began discussing a concept called One Word, in which you choose a word to guide you in the coming year. I had heard about this before but never intentionally chosen my own word at the beginning of the year. My word always seemed to come to me mid-year. Now, I wondered if I should choose a word for 2016 as the year began.

I wanted a pretty word like grace or bravery or joy. A word that didn't need a lot of explanation, a word that would roll off the tongue effortlessly. None of the pretty words would stick. So, I waited. One night between Christmas and New Year's Eve, I was driving home to my apartment from Mom's house. As I drove, I ran through a list of possible words in my mind, but none of them fit. Finally, I half-prayed that God would reveal the word I needed. Within minutes a word came to my mind. *Unbound. Unbound?* I was a little puzzled by this word that seemed unusual. *You mean "free"? It means the same thing, just a little prettier, a little more palatable on the tongue.* Here I was, questioning the higher power who dropped this word in my lap. *No? Unbound. Okay. But why "unbound," specifically?*

I didn't get an answer that night. A few days later, an image from the Bible came to mind: Lazarus standing outside his tomb, having been called back from death by Jesus himself, ragged strips of cloth unraveled from his body. And just days after this, a friend had written these words to me: "I can imagine you tossing off the ropes that bind and taking flight."

Pulling my Bible off the bookshelf, I turned the pages to the gospel of John to read about Lazarus. The passage is as follows:

"Then Jesus, again groaning in Himself, came to the tomb. It was a cave, and a stone lay against it. Jesus said, 'Take away the stone.' Martha, the sister of him who was dead, said to Him, 'Lord, by this time there is a stench, for he has been dead four days.' Jesus said to her, "Did I not say to you that if you would believe you would see the glory of God?" Then they took away the stone from the place where the dead man was lying. And Jesus lifted up His eyes and said, 'Father, I thank You that You have heard Me. And I know that You always hear Me, but because of the people who are standing by I said this, that they may believe that You sent Me.' Now when He had said these things, He cried with a loud voice, "Lazarus, come forth!" And he who had died came out bound hand and foot with grave clothes, and his face was wrapped with a cloth. Jesus said to them, 'Loose him, and let him go.'"[1]

Lazarus had been dead for several days, buried in the darkness of the tomb. But when Jesus beckoned, he emerged from his grave, bound in grave clothes that his friends had to loosen. They had helped him become unbound. *Unbound.* Alive again. Free. Called back to life from death and darkness.

The symbolic parallels between my own story and Lazarus' were startling to me. But at the same time, the word *unbound* made a lot of sense. Since 2013, I had been bound by depression, anxiety, and a total loss of self-worth. I spent two long years in the darkness, buried in shame and sadness. Then, by some miraculously divine intervention, the universe had brought me not just one or two new friends via #the4500 but dozens of them. Reading *Daring Greatly*, meeting Anna in my dream, chatting with her on the phone, and gradually stepping out of the shadows in the Facebook group were reflective of how I was being beckoned to come back to life. And my friends were eagerly waiting to rip off those grave clothes that were tightly bound.

Just a few days after unbound came to me, I read a section entitled "It Was for Freedom" in *Think Differently, Lead Differently* by Bob Hamp. In this section, Hamp relates the truth that freedom comes when the Spirit of the Lord is present and the reality that, often, we become prisoners to thinking that freedom comes from the absence of a behavior or thought pattern:

"The Bible is very clear that freedom is not the absence of something; it is the presence of Someone...Where the Spirit of the Lord is...there is freedom. Freedom is not about the control of impulse and behavior; it is about the fulfillment of identity and destiny. Your identity and destiny cannot be restored apart from the presence of God on Earth. Freedom is about being restored to live life as the man or woman God created and redeemed you to be...it is about unleashing the good things for which you were made." [2]

Having been bound in the prison of depression, anxiety, disbelief, and shame since the Gallaudet incident, every expression of this freedom was stifled. My words, written and spoken, were bound. My mind was bound. My faith was bound. My relationships were bound. My hands, and the language I dearly loved, were bound. My calling was bound. I was bound, tethered by the lies that constantly told me I had failed and was worthless. The weight of the grave clothes was suffocating me.

But since September, I was slowly unwinding the grave clothes, with the help of #the4500, Bob Hamp's teaching, and a tentative hope that I could still trust myself to hear God speak to me. I was becoming unbound. My words were no longer locked away in silence. My mind was no longer held hostage by fear. And I was learning how to be vulnerable with people who had earned the right to hear my story.

On December 28, 2015, I commented on a post about our words for 2016 in #the4500 and said my word was "unbound." Later that afternoon, I was listening to some of Bob Hamp's old podcasts while cleaning my apartment. Because I was moving from room to room and not actively listening, I knew I would probably need to go back and listen again to really hear what he was saying. So, I was quite surprised to find myself sitting on my bedroom floor, sudden tears rolling down my cheeks during an episode titled, "A Kingdom Parable." I stopped what I was doing and listened to Hamp:

"...your dad is so glad you're home...whatever's been asked of you, whatever you're called to do, isn't so that you can perform so an angry, rigid dad would be happy with you, finally. He's saying this: 'Hey, come discover who I made you to be. Put your hand to it. Stand up and speak it, do it. The things that are in your heart to do, the things that make the fire leap up in your chest. Don't shy away from them. Somebody once told you that it's not true about you, but something inside of you knows it is. Freedom isn't where we finally stop the bad stuff...freedom is when you can become the person you're created and redeemed to be. All of those other things are just obstacles." [3]

I was overcome with emotion, sprawled face down on the floor, my tears saturating the beige beneath me. Am I really <u>not</u> a huge disappointment to God? Am I really capable of hearing him for myself? Was Pastor C wrong to tell me not to go to Gallaudet? These questions came to mind in quick succession. I grabbed a notebook from my nightstand and began journaling, writing the answers as they came to mind. I knew that ASL lit a fire in my chest, and had for a long time: why else would I have written my thesis and course proposal as a college undergrad? It was something I believed in wholeheartedly. But someone who I was taught had spiritual authority over me had declared otherwise, unraveling the threads that held that belief together.

In hindsight, I also believe this quote from Bob's podcast struck a chord deep in my soul because of the image of a father and child he used in this parable. When Pastor C told me I would get hurt if I went to Gallaudet, he wrapped those damaging words in a false sense of

familiarity by also saying that he loved me like a daught,
And since I had grown up in a home where my father was
physically present but emotionally absent, that void was
primed to be filled. I was an easy target for being
persuaded that Pastor C had my best interests at heart.
While I don't know what his motives were in telling me
those things, I now know that our very distant relationship
as pastor and congregant did not grant him the right to
express such a baseless claim on my life, much less tie it
to a close personal relationship that did not exist.

So, when I heard Bob say that God wasn't disappointed
in me for failing to do what lit a fire in my soul by not
going to Gallaudet, the sense of relief that flooded me was
understandably overwhelming. Still lying on the floor, I
wrote all the things that were bubbling up inside me.
Finally, I stopped writing and laid my head down again,
my forehead resting on the edge of the notebook. The last
thing I had written was the word "UNBOUND" in capital
letters. I lay there in silence, taking deep breaths, soaking
in the calm I felt after the rush of emotion I experienced.
Within a few minutes, I heard a still, small voice in my
mind: "I am releasing you." *Unbound.*

Chapter 6:

Snowpocalypse

Shortly after New Year's Day, we were discussing our words for 2016 in #the4500. One of the members came from a Jewish heritage and was offering to make custom jewelry engraved with our words if we were interested. She would engrave the words in English, Hebrew, or both. I emailed her immediately and ordered a bar necklace with "unbound" engraved in both languages. The necklace arrived a couple weeks later. Accompanying the necklace was a card that had the Hebrew translation of "unbound": "stretched through the teeth from human strength to divine strength." Suddenly the word's already weighty meaning became heavier. *If this is the word that*

represents this year, what in the world is it going to hold?
I was almost afraid to ask. But I was also looking forward
to the things that were already in motion.

On Christmas Eve 2015, I bought my plane tickets for
Splendid in the Hills. The retreat would take place April
28- May 1, 2016 in the hill country a few hours outside of
Austin. Anna had suggested I fly into Dallas on
Wednesday, April 27, so she could pick me up. I would
stay at her house that night, and we would travel to Austin
the next day. I thought that was a great plan and agreed.
My trip to Texas was definitely something I was looking
forward to in the months ahead. Another was my first in-
person meetup with a member of #the4500.

Five days later, I posted a blog about my word for 2016,
which included a quote from Bob Hamp. Anna tagged
Bob when I shared the post on Facebook. He shared the
post on his own page, amplifying my words beyond my
tiny audience. The next morning, I woke up to more
notifications on my blog than I had ever seen before.
While it only increased my readership by a few hundred
people, it was a huge increase from my handful of regular
readers, most of whom were part of #the4500. I was
shocked to know that my writing resonated with a wider
audience.

Then, one morning in January, I was at work when a text
from Anna appeared. While my students were at P.E., I
checked her message. "FYI: I AM BUYING TICKETS

TODAY!!!!! We can plan for a meetup on Saturday, January 23!"

Yes! To say I was excited was an understatement. Anna's business trip to Charlotte in October had been cancelled, and we had been disappointed that it delayed our opportunity to meet. But now, we were elated that it was finally going to happen in just two weeks.

Over the next few days, we texted back and forth, making plans for Anna to drive to Greenville Saturday morning, and stay at my apartment that night before driving back to Charlotte to catch her flight the next day. We also planned to have lunch with a handful of women from #the4500 who lived in South Carolina, North Carolina, and Georgia. (By that time, it wasn't unusual for people in the group to travel several hours to meet a #the4500 friend who was traveling nearby. We were pretty invested as a whole.)

In the meantime, I was working on a project for Anna. She had been asked to lead two more launch teams since Ruth's, and needed help putting together a presentation of how she operated her launch teams for one of the publishers. Because she was so busy working her full-time job as well as her new part-time side hustle running launch teams, she asked me to help her with the presentation. This was my first freelance administrative project. I was being paid to use my administrative skills behind the scenes to help a friend who would much rather be working directly with people. Little did we know that this was a glimpse of the future.

The week of Anna's business trip arrived and we continued making plans for our short visit. But early in the week, the weather forecast for the Carolinas grabbed our attention. Winter Storm Jonas was headed for the East Coast; the unusually strong Category 4 snowstorm was scheduled to hit the area on Thursday, January 21. Sure enough, I woke up on Friday morning to the news that school was cancelled due to the several inches of snow glazed with ice that had fallen overnight. Clinging to a tiny thread of hope that we would still be able to meet, Anna and I began adjusting our plans. Not wanting to put pressure on others to travel in hazardous conditions, we cancelled our lunch with the others from the surrounding states. But Anna and I were still trying to figure out a way to meet, if only for a quick cup of coffee before her flight departed Charlotte on Sunday morning. I posted in #the4500 and asked the group to pray that Plan B, or even C, would work out so that Anna and I could finally meet in person. No more snow fell on Friday, the weather was sunny, and the temperature was well above freezing. Still, my apartment complex's parking lot was a solid sheet of ice. There was no way I could get my car out. The situation was similar at Anna's hotel in Statesville, just north of Charlotte. Discouraged, I went to bed that night, preparing myself for the looming disappointment.

The next morning, I posted in the group again, ruminating on one of the things I had read in *Daring Greatly.* Brené Brown explained that joy and disappointment are closely related to vulnerability; when we make ourselves enough to express hope and joy, we risk feeling acutely disappointed when whatever brings us hope and joy is threatened. She says, "foreboding joy [is] the paradoxical dread that clamps down on momentary joy."[1] I was definitely feeling that sense of dismay as I frantically scrolled through weather updates that morning. In reply to my text of lament over my deteriorating plans, my friend and co-teacher, Christine, told me, "Whether or not this weekend happens, it is a victory because you showed up, and that is huge. There was a time not too long ago when you wouldn't have been able to make these plans because it was too far out of your comfort zone." She was right, but I so badly wanted the meetup to happen.

By early Saturday afternoon, Anna and I had decided that our best shot was to meet for coffee Sunday morning, if the ice and snow melted enough for me to drive to Charlotte. But as I thought about that plan, I realized I would need to leave my apartment before the sun had time to warm up and melt any leftover precipitation that had refrozen overnight. Scrolling through my Twitter feed, I saw an update from the SC Department of Transportation stating that the interstate between Greenville and Charlotte was clear. So were the main roads between my apartment and the interstate. My apartment was only six miles from the interstate. It was a straight shot to the town where Anna was staying. The main problem was getting my geriatric Honda out of the parking lot. My brain went into full problem-solving mode. *If I can get out of the parking lot, I can get to the interstate. If I can get to the interstate, I can get to Anna's hotel. How can I get there today instead of tomorrow morning?*

I texted Anna and told her about the Plan D that was forming in my mind. She was tentatively optimistic. I, however, was fairly sure that trying to drive my car to Statesville was not a good idea, even if I could get it out of the parking lot. So, I texted my sister to see if she and Mom were up for a little adventure. If they could safely get to my apartment in Mom's four-wheel-drive vehicle, I could meet them at the curb and we could all go to Statesville. It took several hours of pleading to convince them to help me get to North Carolina, but they finally agreed to go. I texted Anna the good news and alerted #the4500 to pray that we could make the trip.

Mom and Jess arrived at my apartment complex late that afternoon and we set out on the two-hour drive. While Mom drove, Anna texted and said that we could stay in her room that night so we wouldn't have to get our own. I was on board with that plan, but Mom and Jess were not; I booked a separate room for them. Surprisingly, I had zero anxiety about meeting Anna in person, even though she was an "internet stranger." In fact, I was "so chill it was weird," as I told Christine at work the next week.

The trip was mostly uneventful once we were on the interstate, until we reached the exit for Anna's hotel. The hotel was only a half-mile off the exit but the frontage road was a sheet of ice. It was already dark and to say that Mom, who was already nervous about this whole excursion, was not thrilled about navigating the slick road to the hotel is a gross understatement. But she did. By the time she parked the car in the hotel's icy parking lot, the tension in the car was palpable. Mom's nerves were shot; Jess was not so happy either. Trying not to let their frustration diminish my excitement, I grabbed my backpack, opened the car door, and gingerly stepped onto the ice. Mom and Jess were taking their sweet time getting out of the car, so I left them and headed toward the entrance to the hotel.

Entering the lobby, my eyes scanned the room for the face I knew only by her profile picture. Sitting across the room, her head bent toward her phone, was the soul-sister I had waited months to meet face-to-face. I stopped at the front desk to check-in and get the key to Mom and Jess's room. Anna glanced up; I caught her eye and waved my hand in the air. Bounding out of her chair, she practically skipped across the lobby. She stopped two feet in front of me, bent forward, hands covering her mouth, and squealed with joy. My smile spread so wide it hurt my cheeks. We hugged each other tightly.

"You're real," I breathed. Words failed us and we just stood there, staring at each other.

"I guess you know each other?" The front desk manager's voice broke through our silent awe.

"Yes," Anna acknowledged.

"We do now," I explained, simultaneously.

Mom and Jess stepped into the lobby just then. Enthusiastically, I introduced them to Anna. Then, I handed Jess their room key and we all headed toward the elevators, where we parted ways. Mom and Jess turned down the hallway to get settled in their first-floor room. Anna and I stepped into the elevator, headed up to her room to chat. We snapped a selfie, both of us grinning ear-to-ear, and posted it in #the4500. We were giddy.

A while later, Mom and Jess knocked on the door. We all sat up late talking and getting to know Anna. Though they weren't yet friends on Facebook, Jess had brought one of her scrapbooks filled with pictures from her European travels to show Anna. At one point, Anna picked up a thick stack of papers from the desk.

"I have something exciting to show you."

She held up the papers and said, "This is the publishing

contract for my book. I just signed it and can't say anything about it on social media because the publisher doesn't have a signed copy yet."

"Eek!" I squealed, leaning closer as she handed it to me. "This is super exciting!" I couldn't believe the timing of everything that was happening.

Around midnight, Mom and Jess returned to their room. Anna and I stayed up a couple more hours, talking until we could barely hold our eyes open. We woke up early the next morning to talk some more as Anna prepared to leave for the airport. When it was time for her to go, we met Mom in the lobby and took a few more pictures. I followed Anna to her rental car in the parking lot. We hugged tightly and said, "See you later." It wasn't goodbye because we already knew we would see one another in April. As I turned to walk back into the lobby, my heart was full. Meeting Anna was just wonderful in real life as it had been in my dream. Not even Snowpocalypse had been able to prevent us from finally being friends in real life.

Chapter 7:

Hard News

After meeting Anna, I began talking about #the4500 and how it had changed my life more frequently. As we had left Anna's hotel room that Sunday morning, I told her I was still taking wobbly baby steps toward my bravery.

"Oh, we're past baby steps," she observed.

"Yeah, I guess this is more like jumping off a cliff," I conceded.

"Exactly," she agreed.

My blog became a public journal of the events that were

taking place. I felt as though I had crossed the chasm from lifelessness to fully alive. My virtual life and in-person life began to merge instead of being separated. I was relieved that Jess and Mom had met Anna, too, before I went to Texas for Splendid.

The first weekend of February brought another new opportunity. I don't remember the first time I heard about IF:Gathering, whether it was Jen Hatmaker's Facebook page or another author's blog, but I was intrigued. When people began talking about it in #the4500 in October 2015, I decided I would register for IF:Local. Each year, the live IF:Gathering in Austin, TX is simulcast to partner locations all over the world. The closest one to me was forty-five minutes away.

My car rolled to a stop in the parking space across the street from the red brick building studded with stained glass shortly after work that Friday evening. I shifted the gear stick into park, turned off the ignition, and took a deep breath. *What are you doing here? Turn the car back on. Leave. You don't have to go in.* Grabbing my phone, I summoned my tribe of internet friends to bolster my courage: "I'm sitting in my car outside the church. Somebody tell me to get my butt out of the car and in the door." They immediately did: many of them. I sat for a few more minutes, heart pounding, feeling nauseated. I knew no one inside the building. But I felt compelled to be there that weekend. I opened the door and stepped out of the car.

Getting out of that car was not what I wanted to do. Running the other way seemed like a more appealing option. But I got out of the car anyway. My steps were unsure and my heart was racing as I walked in the door and joined the registration line. I picked up my name tag and my name was checked off a list. Accounted for, I turned to find a seat at one of the round tables that were spread across the room. A room full of strangers is an introvert's least favorite environment. Sliding into a chair at an empty table in the middle of the room, I pulled out my notebook and tried to look busy and at ease. Eventually, a few others joined me at my table. At one point, a woman from the table in front of me came over and introduced herself because she'd noticed my name and had an uncommon name herself. Then the event started and I relaxed a little.

That first evening session was hard. I felt completely vulnerable and exposed, never entirely comfortable, though hearing author Jo Saxton speak was delightful as she's both wise and hilarious. And by the end of the night, tears were streaming down my face. I went home exhausted and unconvinced that I'd actually make myself return for the all-day Saturday session. In fact, I didn't decide I was going back until an hour before the event started the next morning. I am so glad I did.

Walking into the building Saturday morning, I stopped by the registration table to pay for lunch. Standing there at the table were two women. They moved aside as I approached the table. The woman sitting at the table looked familiar to me and I realized that her son was in the therapy program affiliated with my school. I didn't know her, personally, but I knew who she was. I told her I needed to pay for lunch.

"My name is Ticcoa. I was here last night," I said as she took my cash and found my name on her list.

As soon as my name was out of my mouth, one of the older ladies standing to the side gasped and turned to face me.

"That's such a beautiful name!" she gushed. "It sounds Native American. I love Native American stuff. What does it mean? Where did it come from!?"

I swear I must have looked at her like a deer caught in headlights. Her hands were on my shoulders, rapidly firing these questions at me, and I was struggling to keep up. I offered answers as best I could, hoping they were intelligible. She really was quite lovely about it all; I was just stunned out of my introverted shell.

After a few minutes, she let me go, and I slunk off to the same table I'd sat at the night before, knowing the women who'd sat there the night before weren't attending that day. While I sat there, waiting for the session to begin, I posted on Twitter: *My name forces me out of hiding. Darn name tags.* A few minutes passed and one of the women at the table in front of me waved me over, inviting me to sit with them. So, I moved to their table. There was an empty chair to my left, a pile of belongings on the table in front of it. Just as the session began, the woman who loved my name, Mary Carol, came and sat by me. I smiled, feeling like I had made an instant friend. As the day progressed, it was apparent that the five women seated at this table — Susan, Mary Carol, Donita, Wendy, and Lisa — were close friends. They welcomed me into their circle with more warmth than I could have hoped for that day.

One of the scariest, most beautiful things about IF:Gathering is that during each session, there is a time of guided discussion that is only effective if you're willing to be real and get a bit vulnerable. Through one of these questions, I was able to share my story of the last year with these women, including my involvement with #the4500 and my upcoming trip to Splendid in the spring. When I told these women — who I had only known for a few hours — that I was flying alone for the first time, they immediately asked for the dates, promising to pray for me, and writing down their names so I could find them on Facebook. Susan, who was also busy as one of the event co-hosts, came and sat down with us as I ended my story, and heard me describing #the4500 as "the best 'no' ever." She asked if I had ever read Lysa TerKeurst's book, *The Best Yes.* When I said no, but it was on my list of books to read, she fetched a copy of it from a nearby table and handed it to me: "It's yours, from the church."

A year before IF:Local 2016, I was begging God for community, for soul-deep friendships. I was so caught up in and sick of the comparison game that I was ready to quit social media. But then I got the best "no" from Jen Hatmaker's publisher about her launch team, and found a crazy bunch of girls on Facebook and Twitter who banded together to create a virtual community that grew into something more special than any of us could have imagined. Before #the4500, I never would have considered going to IF:Local alone. But the power of community and our sisterhood made me braver and more courageous, and showed me that I was not alone in my struggles.

The remainder of February was comparatively uneventful than the past few months had been, with the exception of the brilliant idea my two middle siblings—Jess and our brother Josh—presented to me in early March: a matching or coordinating sibling tattoo. Jess presented their case via text message:

"So, Josh and I have been talking...what are your thoughts on sibling tattoos?"

Her question was followed by the cheesy-grin emoji. I shot back a text of twenty-one laughing-to-the-point-of-tears emojis of my own. *Did they not know me at all? My aversion to needles is strong. I didn't even get my ears pierced until I was twenty-seven years old. And they wanted me to get a tattoo? Nope.*

"COME ON!!!" she replied.

"I thought Josh was getting a fam tattoo, not the whole fam is getting tattoos!" I texted. Before she could reply I began probing for information. "Like one design for all? Or complementary designs?" I asked, quickly followed by a disclaimer. "Do not read my curiosity as consent."

"Yeah, he was, but then we started talking about sibling tattoos and he likes the idea," she explained. "It would be small! Do it!"

"What kind of tattoo, though?" I asked, still very resistant to the whole idea. "If I'm permanently inking my body, I want to know what I'm putting on it. Why am I even discussing this?"

"Ermagherd," Jess replied exasperated by my resistance and lack of enthusiasm. "We just wondered if you would even consider it."

"I will consider it with the teeny tiniest bit of consideration," I relented, still not convinced. "I can't believe I'm saying this."

Jess made one last-ditch effort to convince me.

"If you won't do it, we'll probably just kick you out of the family." She was ruthless.

A few days later, she sent me a few designs she and Josh had found on the internet that incorporated our first initials, which were T (me) and three Js (Jess, Josh, and our youngest brother Jordan). We bantered back and forth, negotiating which design we each preferred but never agreeing on one that felt just right. And I still wasn't committed to the idea. I figured if I let them talk about it long enough, they would eventually forget about it and let me off the hook. The subject provided plenty of good-natured sibling arguments and teasing that was typical of our playful dynamic.

But Friday, March 11, 2016 marked a shift in the lightheartedness. There are moments that etch themselves in your mind's eye, for better or worse. That day brought one of those moments.

I was on the playground, watching my kindergarten and first grade students at recess when my phone alerted me to an incoming text message. I looked down at the screen and saw a message from Jess: "I know what I have. Do you want to know now or later?"

I knew she had recently been to the doctor but as far as I knew, Jess was either dealing with an ulcer, a hernia, or a gluten allergy. That's the response I expected when I texted back, "You tell me. Do I want to know now or later?"

A few minutes later, her answer appeared on the screen: "Pseudomyxoma peritonei. It's a rare form of appendix cancer."

My brain scrambled to make sense of the unpronounceable words. I felt my breath leave my lungs as the crushing weight of disbelief hit my chest. In a daze, I stared at the string of letters and put my hand on the column of the play structure to steady myself. Before thinking better of it, I copied the words to the internet browser and searched for the meaning behind the medical jargon. PMP was a terrible disease with a grim prognosis, and my twenty-nine-year-old sister was now facing it. The blood drained from my face.

"What's wrong? Are you okay?" Christine, who was standing nearby, walked over as I slowly lowered myself to the bench beside me, still staring at my phone.

I shook my head no.

"Jess just texted me." I whispered. "She has this."

I handed Christine my phone. She read the words and exhaled. Then, she alerted our classroom aide to watch the kids and sat down beside me.

"I'll call the office and tell them you're leaving if you want to go. You do not have to stay." Christine was in action mode, ready to help as best she could.

I texted Jess back and asked if she wanted me to come over, but she responded that she was tired and not up for company. We both knew we needed some space to process the diagnosis.

"No, I need to stay." I told her. "I can't go home to my apartment right now. I will lose it if I leave now." I knew I would fall apart eventually, but I was already heading into the weekend with this monstrous reality and I wanted to delay it as long as possible, even if just for a few more hours.

When we got back to our classroom, I excused myself to the bathroom to pull myself together. I went through the motions of finishing the school day. Numbness was already setting in; there were so many questions running through my mind. Mom, Jess, and I were the only people who knew about the diagnosis.

At home that afternoon, I scrolled to #the4500 and told them about the diagnosis. I knew I could trust this virtual sisterhood with the terrible news my sister had received.

What is said in #the4500 stays in #the4500. And I knew I couldn't carry this burden alone. It was too much. I need to be able to show up for my sister and that also meant having a safe space to process my own emotions. With tears rolling down my face, I read their heartbroken responses and promises to pray. I felt enveloped in their virtual arms as they encircled me with concern.

I spent much of the weekend at Mom's house with Jess. We didn't talk much about the diagnosis. Instead, we watched movies and hung out much like we usually did. I asked a few questions about the illness, then let her take the lead in discussing it. My insides were swirling, though.

The only in-person friend who knew about Jess' diagnosis was my co-teacher, Christine. Our friendship was sturdy enough that we could be real with each other; we had already walked through difficult things together. This devastating development was no exception.

On Monday, I returned to the classroom, glad for the distraction and comfort my students brought. As they were putting together large floor puzzles after lunch, Christine and I discreetly talked about how I was doing. We were on one side of the classroom and the kids were on the other. She sat on one of the low tables and I sat beside her, both of us facing the kids. Our classroom aides were on their lunch breaks.

"I am so overwhelmed," I told her. "I just want to crawl in

a hole and disappear."

"I know this is hard," she said, her voice filled with compassion and concern. "But I also know that you are a strong person and you love your family. You are going to be a light to them in the difficult days ahead."

"Ugh," I moaned, scooting off the table and into a cross-legged position on the floor. "I'm tired of being a strong person."

I flopped backward and laid on the floor, my hands covering my face. The emotional toll was already affecting me. My body felt so heavy; I just wanted to curl up into a ball right there. Christine sat on the table, her eyes wide and mouth agape. After a few seconds, she glanced up at the window and alerted me that our principal was on the way to our classroom. I rolled over and stood up. My meltdown had passed.

When I got home that afternoon, I went to bed and slept for two-and-a-half hours. I awoke to a text from Christine.

"Okay, reality check: you actually laid on the floor of our classroom and rolled over. You MUST be stressed out of your mind."

I sent a string of red-faced, embarrassed emojis back to her.

"So that wasn't just in my imagination?" I asked.

"No, honey, it wasn't."

The next day, we laughed about the absurdity of my meltdown and the levity of it was a welcome release to the tension. Having someone who I could be myself with was a relief when I felt like I needed to hold it together for everyone else. Christine was the only person I could do that with in real life; everyone else was hundreds of miles away and accessible only by telephone and computer.

In the midst of my newfound aliveness, my family was thrust into the unknowns of terminal illness. I fought to maintain a brave face for my sister and the rest of my family in the weeks that followed, while coming to terms with the suffering Jess was experiencing. As I imagine it does for all who are faced with such news, the initial shock of grief and loss barged into my life without warning. I didn't issue an invitation for grief to ring the doorbell, waltz in, and make itself at home. Still, it showed up unannounced and unexpected.

Two weeks after I got the news of Jess' diagnosis, Anna called to check on me. It was the first time we'd spoken since the diagnosis. After our initial greeting, we sat in heavy silence. Both of us were grappling with the magnitude of the situation. I sat at my desk, staring at a card stuck to my bulletin board. The card that had arrived with my unbound necklace. The card with the Hebrew meaning of unbound. *Stretched through the teeth from human strength to divine strength.*

"I can't believe this is happening," Anna broke the silence.

"I know," I agreed, my voice thin and weary. "It feels like a nightmare."

"There's something I'm grateful for, though," she continued. "I'm so glad you came alive and are walking this road with your whole heart."

"It doesn't feel like I'm doing this in a wholehearted way," I replied. "It feels like my heart is splintered into a million pieces."

"I know," she said. "But you are different than you were even six months ago. You have the tools you need to help you get through this."

At the end of March, I went to Ocean Isle, North Carolina with Mom, Jess, and my youngest brother, Jordan, for Jordan's spring break. My middle brother, Josh, was unable to come due to his work and college schedules. One day, I found myself standing in the waves, eyes locked on the horizon. The water was still quite chilly since it was barely spring. A restlessness stirred in my soul; my heart felt like it was shattered, and salty tears glistened in my eyes hidden beneath sunglasses. As I stood on the Carolina coast, two dear friends in two opposite directions were walking through very hard days. My heart ached to be with both of them, my mind hyper aware of the distance that separated us. And my own family had been slammed with Jess' illness. I was numb and carrying the weight of the world on my shoulders at the same time.

The waves gathered strength and crested all around me, beating themselves against my legs and stomach. My feet shifted in the sand, my muscles aching as they braced against the ocean's continuous attempts to shove me under the water. I stood there until my legs, chilled to the bone, began to give way. Turning, I stumbled back to the shore, where I continued staring at the horizon line.

Though the tension of Jess' illness was thick and the weight of the unknown was heavy, the trip was good for our souls. Jess, Jordan, and I spent one evening on the beach watching the sunset, walking along the shoreline, and taking pictures, all peppered with Jess' sarcasm, Jordan's wit, and my playful intolerance for their shenanigans.

In the weeks following our trip to the beach, I was struggling with whether I should still go to Texas for Splendid. This was especially true after I sat in on Jess' consultation with the surgeon, who scheduled surgery for May 1, the day I was supposed to fly home from Texas. Part of me felt like I should just stay home and focus all my energy on my sister, but I also knew that I needed to go to Splendid for my own well-being. The months ahead were going to be incredibly difficult and I needed to take time to renew my own soul. Being burned out and depleted already would not be helpful to anyone. I was learning that I needed to make sure my cup was full before I started trying to pour into anyone else.

Though I was torn between feeling like I finally had a life of my own and the pressure I felt to be everything my family needed and wanted me to be during these difficult circumstances, I was beginning to learn that the deeply-rooted codependent nature of my familial relationships was unhealthy. Learning to assert and maintain boundaries during a crisis was not ideal. But I also knew that I had to figure out a way to support my sister while also making space for my own life. I was afraid that if I allowed myself to revert to my old ways of thinking and chose the needs of everyone else over my own, I would spiral into the deep dark again. But this time I wasn't sure I would be able to claw my way out. Ultimately, Jess decided to postpone the surgery because she wasn't comfortable with the surgeon or procedure and encouraged me to keep my plans to go to Texas.

Chapter 8:

Welcome to Texas

*"What if I fall? Oh, but my darling,
what if you fly?"*
Erin Hanson

Tuesday

My students and I sat in a circle on the floor after lunch. We were finishing up an activity before going out for recess. They knew about my trip to Texas and that I would not be at school for the rest of the week. A few of them were asking questions about Texas and why I was going. I told them that I was nervous about flying for the first time.

"I've never been on an airplane before," I confessed to the six- and seven-year-olds beside me. We talked about feelings a lot in our classroom, and Christine and I sometimes shared our own with the kids in an age-appropriate manner to model how to deal with a range of emotions. "I'm a little scared."

"Sometimes I'm scared, too, Ms. Ticcoa," one of the boys, Henry, said as he fiddled with a block.

"Yeah, like when I climb on the rock wall at the playground, sometimes it makes me nervous," another boy, Asa, chimed in.

"I just remind him to be brave," Henry offered, matter-of-factly.

"Yeah, Henry tells me to be brave and then I can just climb all the way to the top!" Asa turned to me, excitedly, his eyes bright. "You just have to be brave, Ms. Ticcoa, even if you're scared."

To this day, that conversation is one that comes to mind often. Sometimes I just need to be brave.

That evening, I kneeled on my bedroom floor, clothes strewn around me, one hand pressing the top of my suitcase closed while I pulled the zipper tautly around the middle. I'd already packed, emptied, and repacked my suitcase three times in as many days. To minimize my anxiety as much as possible on my first flight ever, I wanted to travel with only carry-on luggage. With a last shove and pull, the zipper reached the end of its track and the suitcase was securely closed. As I sat back on my heels, my phone rang. A now-familiar Texas area code and number was displayed on the illuminated screen: Anna.

"Hello," I answered, cheerily.

"Hey! I was just thinking, you should bring your Bob Hamp books with you so we can discuss them on the way to the retreat."

"Yeah?" I warily gave my robust suitcase a side-eye glance.

"Yes!" Anna chirped back. "I'm talking about some of his stuff at the retreat, so it would be helpful to talk about what you're learning while we drive."

"Okay, I'll see if I can shove them in my luggage."

We talked for a few more minutes about my flight the next day. Anna offered to be "on call" and walk me through the logistics once I got to the airport in Atlanta. Splendid: Texas was finally here. I was flying in on Wednesday, a day before Splendid began, to stay the night with Anna.

I had felt compelled to be at Splendid since it went live in #the4500 in October of 2015. But while I knew without a doubt that I wanted to attend, six months is a long time to wrestle with the anxiety of leaping so far outside your comfort zone. For me, the decision to fly halfway across the country to spend a weekend with sixty-four internet strangers — only two of whom I had met in person at that point — was entirely out of character.

I was both terrified and excited. So, Anna's offer to guide me through the process of navigating one of the country's busiest airports and getting on the plane before she picked me up in Dallas was much appreciated.

Wednesday

Adrenaline pulsed through my body as I loaded my suitcase into the trunk on my mom's car and climbed in the backseat. She and Jess were making the three-hour drive from Greenville to Atlanta to drop me off at the airport. When we finally arrived at Hartsfield-Jackson International Airport, I unloaded my luggage and started toward the terminal. Jess trailed behind me, snapping pictures and posting them on Snapchat with the caption, "Aw, look at my little traveler." Entering the airport, my senses were immediately overwhelmed. My phone buzzed as I approached the security line. It was Anna, offering moral support from afar.

"You've got this. Breathe. Make sure your pockets are empty, take your shoes off. Electronics in the tray. Breathe. I'll see you in Dallas!"

Mom, Jess, and I stopped short of the line to snap a selfie, then I began slowly weaving my way toward security. My palms were sweaty, and my heart pounded wildly. I reached the front of the line and managed to follow all the steps required to proceed to my gate.

Collecting my possessions in a frenzy, I checked my ticket and set out to find the correct gate. When I got there, I settled in to wait until my flight boarded. For the next hour and a half, I tried to distract myself from the anxiety I felt at the thought of getting on a plane. Eventually, the boarding call rang out on the loudspeaker. Gathering my belongings, I joined the line of people entering the jetway and boarding the plane. I'll never forget the moment I stepped from the jetway to the plane. My stomach lurched as I glanced down and saw the tarmac through the gap between the two surfaces.

Breathe, I silently reminded myself. I lifted my head and made my way down the aisle and selected a window seat. I was not sure yet whether I would peek out the window once we were off the ground, but I wanted to have the option. I settled in my seat and, after listening attentively to the flight attendant give their spiel, I stuck my earbuds in my ears and turned on some music. I'm not sure I moved a muscle as the plane taxied down the runway and climbed into the air. Once we had reached our cruising altitude, I nudged the window open a couple of inches. All I could see were the top of the clouds, so I nudged it open a bit more. Being in the air, on my way to meet so many of the women who had become my friends in the last few months was surreal. For the first time, I was flying, and it was so much more enjoyable than I had expected.

The plane taxied to the gate in Dallas and I texted Anna to let her know we'd landed. I retrieved my luggage and made my way to the airport exit, texting my location to Anna and anxiously looking for a car that matched her description. When she pulled up to the curb, I threw my suitcase and backpack into the backseat and hurriedly jumped in the front seat. Excitedly, we exchanged hellos and hugs across the center console before she navigated through the airport traffic and onto the freeway. I was still shocked that I had made it to Texas.

Anna seemed to have a plan to introduce me to Texas, and our first stop was Torchy's Tacos for lunch. We talked as we ate, and I told her the full story of my failed trip to Gallaudet and the subsequent depression that followed. Though she was listening intently, I noticed that she kept glancing at her watch. Shortly after we finished our meal, she checked the time again.

"Are you ready to go?" she asked.

"Sure," I replied, wondering what was next on the agenda.

We drove a few miles, talking and catching up on each other's lives. I was in the middle of a sentence when she turned into the parking lot of an office complex. Awareness dawned on me as she turned the corner to the lower level offices at the back of the building. I recognized the greenspace behind the building from pictures I had seen on social media.

"Wait. What? Are we...?" I stuttered as I saw the sign: *Think Differently.* Bob Hamp's office. I turned to look at Anna, my mouth agape.

"Are you surprised?" she asked, grinning from ear to ear.

"Yes!" I exclaimed.

"I got here early so you'd have time to pull yourself together. I knew your introverted heart would need to calm down." Anna's voice broke into my thoughts.

She deliberately built in time for me to acclimate to the surprise? How incredibly thoughtful. For most of my life, I have felt like I had to mold myself to the expectations and needs of others rather than honoring my own, so Anna's intentional anticipation of and attention to what I might need in the situation astounded me. I was so appreciative of the obvious care Anna had taken to plan this stop. That moment reiterated to me that the Anna I had met in my dream months ago was, indeed, representative of her true character.

"This is why you told me to bring my books!" The pieces of the puzzle started falling into place.

"Yes, I knew you'd want to get them signed, so I had to think of a reason for you to bring them," she confirmed. "Are you ready?"

I nodded, pulled my books out of my backpack and got out of the car. We entered the building and Anna let the receptionist know we were there for an appointment with Bob. We waited in the lobby for a few minutes. A surreal feeling enveloped me again. I had seen this room online for months as I watched Bob's Tuesday night classes. Now I was standing here.

Bob emerged from the back hallway, greeted us, and ushered us into his office. We visited for a few minutes. Anna and I briefly explained how we had met in a Facebook group. Then she invited me to tell Bob the story about bringing ASL to my alma mater and the Gallaudet incident that I had told her at lunch. So, I told the story again. Near the end, I found myself voicing the beliefs I had internalized as a result of not going to Gallaudet, specifically minimizing my role in my university adding an ASL course to their offerings.

"For a long time, I haven't even been able to give myself credit for being such an important part of the process of starting the program," I explained. "I really haven't been able to own it because I just felt like anyone could've done it."

Anna and Bob glanced at one another.

"Yeah, anyone could have done that," Anna replied with a hint of sarcasm.

"So, you've done all these big things that you didn't think you could do?" Bob followed Anna's question with the question.

"Well, yes," I admitted.

I finally had a realization and could take ownership of the fact that I had a significant role in the fact that thousands of students can now take ASL at NGU. I was passionate and persistent, saw a gap that needed to be filled, took initiative, did the research, and wrote the proposal that set the process in motion. And it was an accomplishment of which I could be — and was — proud.

We talked for a few more minutes, then walked back to the lobby. Bob signed my books, and the three of us took a picture together. Anna and I left the office. Next, she took me to meet her sister, Celia. After Anna introduced us, she told Celia a very brief version of my story. This made the third time I had either spoken it or heard it in the few hours since I landed in Texas.

"You're a powerful woman: a world-changer. Dream big!" Celia directed her words to me as Anna finished the story.

I laughed. *Me, a powerful woman? A world-changer? I don't think so, lady.* I thought these words to myself, yet again minimizing my role in my own experience. At the time, I thought I was exercising humility, a trait "good Christians" were taught to embrace in the church. Really, that perceived humility was hindering me from recognizing the innate abilities I possessed that did, indeed, make me a powerful, world-changing woman. And though I did not yet realize it was happening, I was slowly beginning to grasp that truth.

Chapter 9:

The Splendid Retreat

A hearty knock reverberated through the foyer where Anna and I sat Thursday morning. Our luggage was piled by the door, waiting to be loaded into the car. Anna opened the door and Rachel — a red-headed woman with a gentle yet commanding presence who was part of #the4500 and, serendipitously, lived just a few miles from Anna — entered the house. She and Anna hugged as I waited to the side, excited to finally meet this online friend in person. Rachel turned to me and opened her arms wide, enveloping me in a warm embrace. There was an immediate sense of having known this woman for a long time, just as I had experienced when meeting Anna for the first time. The bonds that were formed in the virtual space of #the4500 reached beyond the internet and gave us the advantage of feeling safe and comfortable with one another when we finally met in person. It was such a beautiful phenomenon to experience.

Our plan was to load Rachel's SUV with our luggage and travel to the Texas Hill Country together but was slightly modified a few days earlier. Now, we were stopping in another city two hours away to meet up with another #the4500 member, Taylor. Anna jumped in the car with Taylor and I stayed with Rachel as we caravanned the rest of the way to the retreat. During the drive, I told Rachel my story. For the fourth time in two days, I related the events that led me into a spiraling depression and battle with anxiety. Rachel listened and offered sympathy and compassion toward my experience, appalled — just as Anna, Bob, and Celia had been — at the declaration Pastor C made when he told me not to go to Gallaudet.

We wound our way through the curvy roads of Texas Hill Country to the mountaintop resort. After checking in, we began unloading the car. Anna and I were assigned to a cabin with two of Anna's friends, Carolyn and Kristen, who had not yet arrived. Discovering that we needed an extra set of sheets in our cabin for a cot, I volunteered to walk back to the office to get them. Cacti-lined gravel pathways connected the buildings on the resort grounds. Short, scraggly trees dotted the property. An expansive, blue sky seemed to stretch for miles over the landscape. Even the aesthetic of Texas was foreign to my Carolina-born-and-bred eyes and I was absorbed in taking it in as I walked, until a bubbly voice broke into my thoughts.

"Ticcoa! Is that Ticcoa!?" A woman stood at the top of the hill, arms waving in the air.

A smile spread across my face as I instantly recognized the voice calling out to me. Mama Lynn. Though we had never met in person, I had heard her voice on videos in the group. Mama Lynn is among the more seasoned members of #the4500, hence the motherly term of endearment many of us have bestowed upon her.

"It *is* Ticcoa!" I yelled back. "Is that Mama Lynn?"

Hugging tightly in the middle of the path, we exclaimed our delight at finally meeting one another in person. This pattern would be repeated as more women arrived at the resort that afternoon. Later, we marveled at how many of us expected the initial meetings would be awkward since we were a group of people who mostly knew one another only online. Yet, again and again, women arrived and were greeted as though we had been friends for decades. We already knew so much about one another's lives from the deep (and sometimes silly) conversations that unfolded in the group. Established connection and understanding allowed us to skip the discomfort of getting-to-know-you small talk, which was a dream for this introvert.

Dinner that night was scheduled at a restaurant in a small nearby town. As we drove down the mountain that evening, I was full of excited anticipation because I knew that a few women were driving straight there from the airport. Among them was Kelli. She and I had formed a fast friendship when I came out of hiding in #the4500. We were both teachers; our siblings were similar in many ways; and we understood and held space for each other on countless occasions. I could not wait to meet her.

We pulled up to the restaurant on the town square and piled out of the car. I followed the group through the door, caught in a bottleneck of women squealing and hugging one another. My eyes scanned the crowd, searching for the face I knew so well from the internet. The bottleneck began to part and I saw her. Kelli. We made contact and I walked straight to her. Enveloping each other in our arms, tears in our eyes, we whispered, "Hello." Hugging her for the first time will always be a memory I treasure. Our arms around one another, we stood together as women continued to arrive.

Soon, we were all assembled, filling half of the small restaurant with our group. Seated at a long row of tables pushed together, among a cacophony of delighted laughter and deep conversation, I marveled at the chain of events that brought me to Texas, to this group of women, to #the4500, to Splendid. My heart was filled to the brim with gratitude.

That night, I rode with Kelli back to the resort and followed her to her cabin to visit before we parted for the night. While sitting in her room, I recounted my story, telling it for the fifth time since I arrived in Texas.

On Friday morning, Anna, Kristen, and I drove down to breakfast with Taylor. The road from the resort to the main road was half-paved, half gravel and, because Taylor was slightly generous with her speed, the car bounced rather clumsily down the mountain. (We still joke about careening down the mountain that morning!) With one hand on the dash in front of me to brace myself, I twisted around in the front passenger seat so I could see Anna and Kristen in the back seat. Anna was telling us a story about an exercise she participated in at another retreat she'd attended several years before.

"So, one day during the retreat, we were given a map of the ranch and some instructions with journaling prompts and told to spread out on the five-hundred-acre property," Anna explained. "Like the Israelites wandering the wilderness, we were supposed to wander the ranch from dawn to dusk. Armed with a map, my watch, some water,

Gatorade, a pen, and my journal, I walked further and further from the main buildings. I paid close attention to landmarks on the map so I would know how to get back at the end of the day."

I shifted in my seat to get a better view of Anna, who was in the seat directly behind me as she continued telling her story:

"Late afternoon approached, and I began to worry about being able to find my way back. I didn't want to be one of the stragglers who got lost. Then, a thought came to me: *you don't have to go back the same way you came.* And as I pondered that thought, I knew that not only was I not going back to the main part of the property the same way I had come geographically, but that I also was not going back home the same way I had come to the retreat, spiritually."

When she said those words, I felt like I had been jolted by a spark of electricity. The force of the phrase, "not the way you came," struck me because of something my friend, Christine, had said the day before I left for Texas. As we left school that day, she said, "I could never spend a weekend with people I only knew online. You aren't going to come back the same person that you are now." So, when Anna said almost the same thing in the car that morning, I felt seen for the first time in a very long time.

I turned around in my seat. Taylor and I glanced at each

other. I could tell Anna's words had meant something significant to her, too. Anna kept talking, but I was not listening. During breakfast, I couldn't get those five words out of my head: *not the way you came.* When we finished and climbed back into Taylor's car, Anna suggested that I tell Kristen and Taylor my story. So, for the sixth time in less than two days, I recounted the story again.

The Splendid Retreat officially began Friday evening. In our first session, Tracy welcomed everyone, relayed basic instructions for the weekend, and paired us up for an icebreaker game. We were to tell our partner two truths and one lie, and she would guess which statement was the lie. Games like this are introverts' hell, so I was less than thrilled to participate. I was paired with Amanda, who was also our worship leader for the weekend. After the game, we were split into small "Family Time" groups: three or four women with one of the Splendid planning team members as the group leader. Anna led the group I was in along with Taylor, Megan, and Melissa, who arrived later that evening. We sat on the floor in the corner of the conference room and exchanged brief introductions. Then, Anna looked at me, and I knew what was coming.

"If we're going to be a family this weekend, I should tell Megan the story, shouldn't I?" I asked.

"Oh, a story? I want to hear it!" Megan encouraged as

Anna and Taylor nodded.

For the seventh time in two days, I told my story. When I got to the part where Pastor C told me not to go to Gallaudet, Megan's eyebrow furrowed, she sat up straighter with an air of righteous indignation about her. Like everyone else, she was incensed on my behalf at his bold, unsolicited declaration. After dinner, we walked over to the resort dining room for dinner. We were enjoying our meal, chatting and laughing, when Amanda walked over to our table and stopped at the corner where I was sitting.

"Tracy wanted me to ask if you would be willing to sign during worship this weekend?" she asked.

I almost choked on my food. My breath caught in my throat. My chest felt like it had been hit with a brick, and my stomach dropped. I looked at her with wide eyes, managing to indicate that I needed to think about it.

"I'll send you my playlist so you can see what's on the agenda," Amanda offered.

She returned to her table and I looked at my tablemates in shock. They were already excitedly agreeing that this was an amazing opportunity. I was not convinced.

"Breathe," Anna reminded me.

I took a deep breath, then another.

"So, is this a 'hell, yes'?" Anna asked, making a reference to one of Jen Hatmaker's signature quotes.

"No, no, it is not," I replied adamantly.

I began listing all the reasons why I should not, could not, and would not do this. It had been three years since I signed in front of people other than my students; I had forgotten too many signs; my fluency was diminished; I wasn't qualified to help lead worship. Anna, Megan, and Taylor shot down every one of my excuses.

"So, this is a 'hell, yes'?" Anna inquired again.

"Not yet. I need to know what's on her playlist for tonight," I replied.

I pulled up the list on my phone. The four songs for that night were the ones I knew best on the entire playlist, one of which I had been playing repeatedly for the past few months. *Fine.* My resistance was faltering.

"I can't get up there and sign in front of people dressed like this," I made a final attempt at an excuse, gesturing to my t-shirt and shorts. (Old Southern Baptist traditions have deep roots.) But even I knew I was grasping at that point.

"See, you're supposed to 'be the light,'" Megan stated, "Your shirt says so!"

"Okay, I'm not saying 'yes' yet, but I'm going to change clothes in case I decide to do this," I told them as I stood up from the table and took a step toward the door. To my surprise, the three of them got up too, and walked out the door behind me. That simple action showed me that I was not alone. My friends had my back and were there to support me.

"You're glowing!" Anna exclaimed as we walked out of the building. "Your smile is from ear to ear! I love this!"

"It is?" I asked, confused. I felt like the panic I was experiencing on the inside was surely evident on my face. I did not even realize I was smiling until Anna brought it to my attention.

We walked back to my and Anna's cabin where I changed clothes. Megan and Taylor sat on one bed while Anna and I sat on the other bed. I pulled up the song I knew best on my playlist and began to sign, trying to make sure my hands still remembered what they were supposed to do after being still for so long. The four of us got quiet, then Anna began massaging my shoulders to ease the tension that had built in them. A few minutes later, I felt her place one hand on top of my head and start playing with my hair with the other. I sat there with my eyes closed, focused on regulating my breathing and calming my racing heart, while Taylor and Megan quietly sang. The atmosphere in the room shifted to a peaceful calm. Finally, I knew I was going to sign during worship that night. There was something wholly sacred about that moment that I will never forget.

At about the same moment the song ended, our roommate, Carolyn, walked in the door to get her notebook. It was time to go to the conference room for the evening session. Taylor and I were walking slightly ahead of Megan, Carolyn, and Anna. Taylor put her arm around my shoulders and offered encouragement, "This is a safe place. This is a place where you can do this."

Behind us I could hear Anna and Megan giving Carolyn a brief synopsis of what was happening. When we got to the conference room, I let Amanda know that I would join her at the end of her set for the closing song. We agreed that she would not call me up; I would just move to the front when she began playing the song.

Throughout that session, I sat on the floor in the back corner of the room, writing all the things that were pouring into my mind — things the Holy Spirit had spoken to me over the past few months, the reasons why I should and should not be doing this — just all the words. When the session began to close, I quietly made my way to the front row. My heart was pounding. Amanda went to the keyboard and I stood up, took a couple steps forward, and turned to face the crowd. She started playing and singing; I closed my eyes and started signing. And it was so hard. My hands kept fumbling, though no one in the crowd probably noticed, feeling awkward and uncooperative.

Ticcoa Leister

But I did what I had been asked to do.

Chapter 10:

You're Not Going Back the Way You Came

Standing at the rear of Anna's car, by a bustling airport curb, we hugged tightly, silently. I'm terrible at saying goodbye. All the words bubble up in my chest, but get stuck in my throat. And really, there aren't enough words. Stepping back, I reluctantly pulled my suitcase out of the trunk, flung my bag over my shoulder. Without making eye contact again, I turned toward the sidewalk and slowly walked away, breathing deeply with each step.

Inside the airport, I paused for a moment to get my bearings, and then headed for the security line, fighting the lump that was forming in my throat and the tears that were pooling in my eyes. My phone vibrated in my hand as I joined the line. I looked down at the text: "You are not going back the same way you came." The lump rose and the tears began to fall, and I heard a small voice in my mind say, "This is not the last time you'll be here...you will be back."

Leaving Texas after Splendid was hard. I felt so at home there. Anna's hospitality, the in-person manifestation of #the4500's online community, the freedom in being myself without the constraints of filling roles I had always filled in the context of family and friends who had known me my whole life, the realization that my story mattered and resonated with other people — all of these aspects of the weekend were a balm to my soul. I did not want to lose the sense of freedom I had gained. But my life back in South Carolina was waiting for me.

From the time Anna dropped me off at the airport in

Dallas on Monday morning, until the time I landed in Atlanta that evening, I cried. I was exhausted in every sense — physically, mentally, emotionally — from the past five days. I had been as fully present and extroverted as I could be at Splendid. Now, I was alone with my thoughts. My perception of myself, of God, and of the women who came into my life through the internet had shifted in ways I couldn't begin to comprehend.

When Mom and Jess picked me up at the airport in Atlanta, I jumped in the car and began relaying my adventures; I had Anna on speakerphone to help me tell my stories. I was gushing with words, talking nonstop for much of the first two hours of our trip back to Greenville. For someone who was usually quiet and reserved, this was completely out of character. But I was so happy and astounded by everything that had transpired, I could not help it. Joy was bursting from my pores.

Over the next few days, I began thinking about going back to Texas someday. Just before Splendid, I had done a random internet search for ASL programs in Texas. This wasn't entirely unusual. Since writing my thesis in college, I had been on the hunt for an ASL-related degree that would fit well with my career objectives, signing skills, and already-held degree. But this time, I found a program that was exactly what I had been looking for: a Master of Science in Education of the Deaf at Texas Woman's University. There was only one caveat: it was a hybrid program. Most classes were offered online, though there were a few classes and practicums that required in-person attendance. But it was only a few miles from Anna's house.

My mind wandered back to this information in the days immediately after Splendid. From my perspective, it seemed like an answer to my prayers and the perfect way to redeem the past few years. A plan to go back to Texas for an extended visit began developing in my brain. Jess was still undecided on whether she would opt for the debulking surgery. And while I felt guilty for thinking about leaving, I also knew I couldn't stop living my life. I had already spent so much time living to make sure everyone else was okay and neglecting my dreams and desires. It was an excruciating position to be in, but I knew that if I did not, at the very least, explore this option, I would be doing a disservice to myself. Even then, I wrestled with making the decision that was best for me.

I had confided in Christine that I felt drawn to Texas for a variety of reasons. A week after I returned from Splendid, I was verbally processing all the obstacles that stood between me and for the summer with her. We sat in our quiet classroom at the end of the school day.

"I just don't know what to do," I lamented. "I feel like this is the opportunity I have been waiting for, but the timing absolutely sucks." Christine turned and looked at me.

"I know it does," she empathized. "But if you're really going to do this, now is the time. If this is really what you feel like you need to do, do it."

"I do feel like this is what I need to do," I said.

"Okay, then, are you just giving lip service to the idea, or are you actually going to act on it? If you wait for the circumstances to be perfect, you won't do it. You will overthink it."

She was right, and I knew it. Her questions and statements cut to the core of me.

"What is happening to my life?" I asked incredulously.

"You're getting a life; you're living your life," she answered.

When I got home from work that evening, I texted Anna.

"I have a question for you," I typed on my phone. "But I don't want you to answer immediately. Think about it first."

"Okay," she texted back. "What's your question?"

"Remember that Deaf Education program at TWU I found back in April?"

"Yes."

"If I were to come to Texas this summer to look for a job and visit TWU, could I stay with you?"

"YES!" Her reply came immediately. "I have an empty room upstairs where you can stay."

Over the next two days, it became apparent that this visit might be longer than I originally anticipated. The lease on our apartment was up in June, so my roommate and I had been trying to decide whether to renew or move. I realized that I had no idea what I would be doing after the summer and couldn't commit to renewing the lease with her. Suddenly, I needed to do something with all my furniture and everything I wouldn't need while I was in Texas. On Thursday night, I met my mom for dinner and told her I was going to Texas indefinitely, but at least for the summer. She was not surprised and said she had thought this was coming. I followed her to her house after dinner to tell Jess. I knew this was going to be hard. Jess was in the kitchen when I walked in.

"Hey, Little Buddy," I said, closing the door behind me. "I need to tell you something."

"You're moving to Texas, aren't you?" she asked, her voice tinged with a mixture of awe and disappointment.

"Yeah," I confirmed, a bit sheepishly.

I knew this was going to be incredibly hard for both of us. Until I'd moved into my apartment a year-and-a-half earlier, we had been joined at the hip. And even then, I was only twenty minutes away and saw her several times a week. The six weeks she had spent in Europe a handful of years before was the longest period of time we had been away from each other since she was born.

After I told Mom and Jess, I called Anna and told her how things were changing, fast. She was excited for me and willing to provide a place for me to stay while I got on my feet in Texas. Suddenly, I had a lot to do in a short amount of time. I gave myself a date by which I wanted to be in Texas — June 11, 2016 — and got to work. At first, I planned to fly to Texas and ship a few boxes of my belongings. Everything else I wanted to keep would go in a storage unit until I knew what my plans were. I told myself I was only going for the summer but was really planning to give myself until November to decide whether I was going to continue living in South Carolina or make a more permanent move to Texas. I chose November as my point of reference because I already knew I would be back in the Carolinas for the Splendid by the Sea retreat, which had been announced just before Splendid in the Hills.

The next hardest task, after telling Jess that I was going to Texas, was telling Christine. My heart ached just thinking about it. We were both saddened that we would no longer be working together.

But, because I wasn't sure of my long-term plans, I knew it wasn't fair to keep her and my principals wondering about whether I would be back the next fall. The responsible thing to do was go ahead and resign. On May 23, 2016, I met with my bosses and gave my resignation. Things were beginning to feel very real.

In the meantime, another unexpected opportunity had arisen. I was scrolling through my Facebook feed one night when I saw that someone had tagged Bob Hamp in a post about a conference where he was speaking the next weekend. The conference just happened to be in a city less than two hours from Greenville. I could not believe I had just met him in Texas and now he was coming to speak in South Carolina. I immediately connected with the conference coordinator and signed up for the conference. A couple days before the conference, Mom decided she wanted to go, too. On Thursday, May 19, I drove to Anderson right after work. I took off the next day of work so I could attend the full day of the conference, so Mom and I drove together. I had listened to a lot of Bob's teaching online and read one of his books already, so this wasn't entirely new material for me. But I had never heard him teach in-person and was excited to be in the audience. On Saturday, we drove separately because I had plans right after the conference ended. After the last session that afternoon, I approached Bob and told him that I was moving to Texas for the summer and would be there in three weeks.

"Wow, lots has happened since I saw you a couple of weeks ago," he mused.

"You have no idea," I answered.

I left the conference and drove to a Cracker Barrel restaurant just outside of Anderson. I was meeting Camille, one of my soul-sisters from #the4500 for dinner. It was our first in-person meetup. I was thrilled and not nervous at all. By this time, meeting internet strangers-turned-BFFs was a normal activity. I got there first and was waiting outside the restaurant when she arrived. We immediately recognized each other and hugged. Over dinner, I relayed what had happened at Splendid. Camille was one of the first people to hear the whole story. Then I told her how I was going back to Texas in a few short weeks.

When I finished talking, I sat fiddling with the butter knife beside my plate. Camille sipped her water. I could tell she was pondering something. She lowered her glass and peered over it at me.

"So, you signed three times at Splendid?" she asked. I nodded and she continued. "Do you know what the number three means in the Bible?"

This time, I shook my head. "No. I used to, but don't remember."

"Confirmation," she said, eyeing me with a raised eyebrow.

"Huh." I stared at her for a second. "Well, I guess that means I'm on the right track, then, doesn't it?" I was astounded by all the little — and not so little — things that were piling one on top of another. These little signposts pointed me in the direction of something bigger than I could envision.

❧

The school where I taught was a small, private school. Our classes were blended grades, so we had most of our students for both kindergarten and first grade. We worked hard to foster a sense of belonging and community in our classroom, not only for the kids but also for the aides who spent time in our room. Saying goodbye to my little classroom family was difficult. During the last week of school, I spent hours sorting through the hundreds of pictures I had taken throughout the year for our annual slideshow. Reminiscing over all the sweet, fun moments we had and knowing I wouldn't experience those moments the following year was bittersweet. I could barely hold back the tears.

On May 26, the last full day of school, Christine and I

kept ourselves busy with final preparations for the end-of-year presentation that would take place the next day, packing up the classroom, and managing the nervous excitement that had our students buzzing. After lunch, Christine asked me to read a book to the kids while she cleaned up from lunch. When she finished, I was still reading. I saw her leave the building out of the corner of my eye and go to her car. She came back and stood outside the door until I finished reading. One of the boys noticed her standing there.

"Oh! Ms. Ticcoa, it's your—" Henry's eyes got wide as he clamped his hand over his mouth. Christine, holding a package behind her back, put a finger to her lips, reminding our students to keep their secret.

"Whew!" Henry lowered his hand and took a deep breath. "Sorry, Ms. Christine. I almost ruined the surprise."

The kids crawled closer to me as Christine moved to put the brightly-wrapped package down in front of me. "Give Ms. Ticcoa some room," she reminded them. They sat back, excitedly waiting for their surprise to be revealed.

"We made something for you to take to Texas while you weren't here last Friday," she explained.

"Aw," I said, touched by her thoughtfulness and amazed that they had kept it a secret all week. Tears instantly stung the corners of my eyes when I unwrapped their gift. It was a black metal photo frame, the kind has clips on bars for the photos. Hanging from wire clips were eleven black-and-white photographs, one for each of my students. Each picture showed a student's hand forming a letter of the ASL alphabet. On the top bar, three little hands held up Y-O-U. The middle bar held A-R-E. Along the bottom bar hung L-O-V-E-D. *You are loved.*

"Oh my gosh," I gasped, my throat raspy with emotion. The kids were moving closer, pointing out which hand was theirs. I looked up at Christine.

"Thank you," I said to her, putting my hand over my heart. "This is the best!"

The next morning, I arrived at school early. When Christine arrived, I was pulling out materials for the day. Our end-of-year program was that morning, followed by our classroom presentation. All of our students, their parents, and other family members would crowd into our classroom; we would hand out awards, tell each student how we had seen them grow over the year, and watch the slideshow, which Christine and I had a reputation for making parents cry during. We were both prepared for tears but knew this year would be even more emotional as our co-teaching relationship ended.

"Don't look at me," Christine said as she put her things away, glancing over her shoulder at me. "If you cry, I'll cry."

"Okay, no eye contact and no crying until after all the festivities," I agreed, making eye contact with her.

The day passed far too quickly. After all of our students left, we sat in the empty classroom for a few minutes and said our goodbyes. I gathered my things and left Academy 3 for the last time. I climbed in my car and pulled out of the parking lot. I had only driven a half-mile before the tears began pooling inside my sunglasses. I stopped at a traffic light, sobbing, and pulled off my sunglasses, frantically wiping at the deluge of tears.

When I got home, I put on my pajamas and went straight to bed, emotionally drained and exhausted. A few hours later, I woke and started crying again as I opened the pile of gifts and cards from my students and their families before going back to bed. The next day was Saturday, and I woke to the reality that I had less than two weeks to clean out my apartment and be ready to move to Texas.

I enlisted Jess's help, and over the next week-and-a-half, we went through every item, paper, and piece of clothing in my possession. The living room was divided into several zones: stuff to donate, stuff to sell, stuff to throw away, stuff Jess was keeping, stuff that I was putting in storage, and stuff that was going to Texas. By far, the donation pile was the largest one. Mom and Jess were going to drive me and my stuff out to Texas, so the going-to-Texas pile was the smallest. I needed to pare down the essentials in order to fit it in Mom's small SUV. We worked endlessly, chatting and listening to Jess's eclectic playlists. Mom and my brothers dropped in occasionally to help, but it was mostly my sister and me alone. We kept #the4500 entertained with our sisterly banter on social media; several of my friends had sent Jess Facebook friend requests and followed her on Twitter, so they loved watching our shenanigans from afar.

I also spent that week meeting my closest friends for coffee or dinner to catch up and let them know I was moving to Texas indefinitely. Every one of them was excited for me, but it was hard to say goodbye again and again.

On Thursday, June 9, 2016, I stood in the doorway and looked around at my nearly-empty apartment. Only my roommate's belongings were left inside. I stepped outside, pulled the door closed, and locked it. I took one last load of my belongings to my storage unit, then headed to Mom's for the night. It was after dark when Mom and Jess were packed for the trip and I began the process of trying to fit their luggage and my belongings into the car. I have never liked puzzles very much, but managed to figure out how to get everything loaded. I slept fitfully on Mom's couch that night, partly because I was excited about getting to Texas and partly because I was nervous about the major transition that was about to happen.

Early the next morning, we set out for Texas. Mom was driving, Jess was in the passenger seat, and I was in the backseat. When we stopped at the gas station, Jess reached into her bag as Mom got out to pump the gas.

"I brought a mascot for our road trip," she announced to me, holding up a green, plastic dinosaur. "I found him at a thrift store and thought he looked lonely."

"Ha!" I laughed. "What's his name?"

"I dunno yet," she said. "What do you think about Monty?"

"Ehh, I don't love it," I responded, knowing she had already decided that was his name.

"Migrating Monty," she said, proudly. She placed Monty in the corner of the dash in front of her. For the whole trip, except for a few brief sightseeing excursions, that's where he stayed.

Our objective for the day was to get to Tupelo, Mississippi early enough to visit Elvis Presley's birthplace. Jess had been obsessed with Elvis since she was six years old and remained a huge fan. The prospect of visiting his birthplace and museum was one of the reasons she decided to come on the trip. We stopped there in the early afternoon and spent a couple of hours touring the house, museum, and grounds. Then, we headed a bit further west to stop at William Faulkner's home in Oxford. This was my gratuitous literary stop for the trip. I am unashamedly obsessed with author homes and historic literary sites, and was determined to add this one to my list of places I have visited. We arrived at Rowan Oak as the sun was beginning to set. It was just a few minutes after the house closed for tours. I was disappointed, but also glad just to be able to roam around the grounds for a while. While Jess and I were taking pictures of the trees that surrounded the house, Mom had noticed the docent come outside to sweep the porch. She struck up a conversation with him and, in a few minutes, called for me and Jess to come over. The docent had graciously offered to let us do a quick walkthrough of the house! I was thrilled, oohing and aahing my way through the hallways.

We stayed in Jackson, Mississippi that night and continued our journey further west the next morning. We made a brief stop at the Louisiana state line to gaze at the mighty Mississippi River, which I appreciated because of its association with Mark Twain. Then we hopped back in the car and made our last push toward Anna's house. We hit Dallas at rush hour, which was not a pleasant experience for Mom, who was driving, but quite entertaining for Jess and I as we tried to calm her down.

Twelve-lane highways and my mother do not mix well!

We arrived at Anna's house at 9:00 p.m. Mom parked by the curb in front of the house, and Anna met us outside, excitedly welcoming Mom and Jess to her home. Her son, Caleb, was there as well. He and Jess had followed each other on Snapchat for a few months and he wanted to meet her. Anna took us inside and showed Mom and Jess her bedroom, where they would be sleeping. Anna insisted on sleeping on the couch so that Jess would not have to navigate the stairs.

When Mom, Jess, and I met Anna back in January, Jess had still been in bed when Anna left for the airport that Sunday morning, and couldn't be persuaded to get up to take a picture with her. Later, when we were in the car on the way back home while Anna was sitting in the airport awaiting her flight, she and Jess were bantering on Twitter. Anna lamented not having a picture with Jess. Jess countered with a snarky remark about Anna being in her fan club and told her she would send her a headshot to hang in her house. Anna then playfully named herself the president of Jess's fan club. So, when I came to Texas in April for Splendid, Jess sent a gift for Anna: an eight-by-ten-inch headshot, autographed for the "president of her fan club." Anna howled with laughter, her eyes glistening with tears when she opened the envelope.

As Anna ushered Mom and Jess into her bedroom, they passed a tiny alcove in the hallway. Anna paused and dramatically used her hands to gesture to the decor there. A small white dresser held two tall, white pillar candles that were lit. Just above the candles, Jess's headshot hung in a frame on the wall.

"See?" Anna asked proudly. "I AM the president of your fan club!"

Jess laughed and shook her head. The next morning, she tweeted a picture of the alcove: "Wake up in TX in a home I've never been in, and a person I've only met once has this lovely Jessica shrine." Anna had won her over.

On Monday morning, June 13, 2016, I walked out to the car with Mom and Jess as they prepared to leave.

"You have good people here," Mom told me as we hugged. "I'm glad."

Rachel and Julie, another friend from #the4500 who lived in the area, had come over to Anna's the night before to meet Mom and Jess and welcome me back to Texas.

"Yes, I do," I replied.

I watched from the curb as they drove away. When they turned the corner, I walked back inside and laid down on the couch. For the first time in weeks, I had nothing to keep me busy. I had just moved halfway across the country. I had no immediate plans, no car — I had left even that in South Carolina because there was no way my twenty-two-year-old Honda would have survived the trip to Texas — and no job yet. The adrenaline was wearing off and the shock of what I had done was setting in. Anna was working in her home office that afternoon and I stayed on the couch for the rest of the day. Because she knew I was overwhelmed and needed a significant amount of time alone as an introvert, Anna did not speak to me for a full twenty-four hours after Mom and Jess left.

Slowly, I adjusted to life in Texas. Over the next few months, I found a part-time job as a behavioral therapist. I was able to attend in-person classes at Think Differently. Anna and I were busy with book launches; she hired me to do a few more small projects here and there. In late August, Anna was in the midst of editing her memoir, which was due to release the following spring. One night, we were sitting in the living room. I was laying on the couch reading; Anna was in the recliner, combing through edits from her publisher on her laptop. Periodically, she sighed deeply. I knew she was working to meet a deadline that night and had a lot of editing left.

"Ugh," she moaned. "I'm so done looking at these edits."

I sat up, facing her.

"Hand me your laptop," I said. I knew the edits were mostly questions that she needed to answer in the manuscript, adding more information and clarifying some details.

"I'll read the questions, you talk, and I'll type," I told her.

"Deal," she said as she handed me the laptop.

Suddenly, I had a new part-time, freelance job: one I had only ever dreamed of having. Over the next two months, we finished the edits for Anna's book. And as Anna was hired for an increasing number of book launches, I took on more of her administrative tasks. We found that we were well-suited to work together, each of our respective skills complementing the other's.

In October, Mom and Jess came to Texas for a long weekend to attend a cancer conference and see if they could get a consultation with a surgeon who had experience treating PMP. I picked them up from the airport and took them to their hotel. While Mom attended sessions that weekend, Jess and I spent time together both at the hotel and Anna's house. Jess's health was far worse than it had been in June and it was startling to witness. I could tell she was weary, both in body and spirit.

In early November, I was writing a blog post and stopped to ponder the fact that my self-imposed milestone of five months in Texas was fast approaching. I realized that I did not want to move back to South Carolina in a few weeks; I wasn't finished with Texas yet, and I did not think Texas was finished with me.

I returned to the Carolinas for Splendid by the Sea. April, another one of my friends from #the4500, picked me up at the airport in Atlanta and I spent the night at her house. The next morning, we picked up three other women who were also attending the retreat and drove to the North Carolina coast. When we crossed into South Carolina and passed the exit to Greenville, April reached over and patted my knee.

"Welcome home," she said. It was the first time I had seen my home state since June. Texas didn't quite feel like home yet, and upstate South Carolina enveloped me with warm familiarity. Still, I did not feel like it was time to come back for good.

After Splendid by the Sea, I drove back to Statesville with Anna, who had flown to North Carolina a few days before me. Now she was staying in town on business for another week, and I was going to Mom's house for two weeks to spend the Thanksgiving holiday with my family. Those two weeks were both difficult and good for my soul, not only because it gave me a reality check on Jess's health, but also because I was not the same person I was when I left in June. I did not quite fit the role I always had in our family but wasn't sure yet what my new role was.

I had not come back the same way I had gone.

Chapter 11:

The Texas—
Carolina Divide

By December 2016, Jess's health had declined enough that I quit my job and flew back to South Carolina for an extended stay through Christmas, at least. I was divided between the two states, embracing my emerging life in Texas and desiring to be close to my sister in South Carolina. I was there for three and a half weeks before returning to Texas just before New Year's Day.

The next week, I interviewed for a job at a nearby preschool, intending to work through March. Then, I would leave to spend April through July with Anna on her book tour. My interview went well and I was offered the job, which I was less than enthusiastic about accepting. I told Anna how I was reverting to a teaching job with less-than-adequate pay.

"I may as well have stayed in SC if I'm just going to work at a daycare," I groaned one day while we were in the car.

"What if you don't have to work in a daycare?" she asked. I looked at her as we stopped at a red light. "You're already working for me. I'll give you a raise and you can just work for me, if you want," she continued. "Unless you just want to teach four-year-olds?"

"No, I would much rather just work for you," I said. "All the things I'm already doing for you are things that I feel are my superpowers. I haven't ever felt like I was putting my degree to work as much as I am now."

"Okay, then you don't have to teach preschool."

Having the flexibility of working for Anna rather than a typical 8-to-5 job also gave me the flexibility to go back to SC as needed without having to negotiate time off. This took a lot of pressure off, though it was still stressful.

In mid-January 2017, Jess went to the ER with shortness

of breath and was admitted by a doctor who was willing to try draining some of the fluid off her abdomen without pressuring her to undergo the entire debulking surgery to remove the affected organs. He was able to drain enough fluid that it provided some relief, but the prognosis was still grim. And now, because the disease had progressed to such a degree that her organs were thickly coated with cancer-filled mucus and her body was so weakened, the doctors were less hopeful that she would make it through and recover from the surgery. The day before the procedure to drain the fluid, I spent hours curled up on the couch beside Anna, sobbing about the entire situation.

While she was in the hospital, Jess's texts to me had portrayed her discouragement. She told me she was ready to have the surgery, asked my opinion on whether she should risk it, and expressed how much she missed me and wished I were there. Once Jess was discharged from the hospital in Charleston, she and Mom drove to an alternative medicine clinic in Myrtle Beach, hoping that treatments there would strengthen her immune system before the surgery.

I flew back to Greenville a week later on Super Bowl Sunday, where our family friends, Eric and Olgui, along with their daughters, Sophia and Emma, picked me up from the airport. We had lunch at Mom's house that afternoon. The next day, my youngest brother, Jordan, and I drove Jess' car to the hotel where Mom and Jess were staying in Myrtle Beach. Each day, Mom, Jess, and I went to the clinic around lunchtime and stayed through the afternoon. Sometimes Mom would leave to run errands or work on her real estate business and I sat with Jess, chatting about surface-level topics. I even read part of Anna's book aloud. By the time we returned to the hotel each evening, Jess was exhausted. On the nights she wasn't too tired, I laid on her bed and watched TV with her or scrolled social media together, catching up on the latest news.

The following weekend, Mom needed to go home to attend to some business, as well as take Jordan back home. Jess and I remained in Myrtle Beach. We were all nervous about Jess's health, well aware that any number of situations that would necessitate me taking her to the ER could arise. I would also be responsible for flushing out the port that had been put in her arm for her treatments each night. Tensions were high, though we all tried to put on our bravest faces.

On Friday, I drove Jess to the clinic. That evening, stubborn "sasshole" that she was, she tried flushing her port herself but she couldn't quite maneuver the way she needed. So, she summoned me.

"Ohh, Da-ko-ta," her sing-song voice rang out, using one of the many nicknames she'd adopted for me over the years.

"Yes?" I asked as I walked through the bedroom door.

"I need help," she said, nodding toward the supplies on the nightstand. I took a deep breath.

"Okay, tell me what to do," I bravely said. I'd watched Mom flush the port several times but was very nervous to do it on my own.

Jess talked me through the whole process, but after trying two or three times, I couldn't get the port flushed. Both of us were getting anxious and frustrated. And I also squirted the ceiling with more saline solution than was necessary while trying to get the air bubbles out of the syringe, but it brought some much-needed comic relief to the tense situation.

Before my fourth attempt, I grabbed my phone off the nightstand and scrolled to the #the4500 Facebook group. I typed a plea for my #the4500 sisters to pray me brave and the port flushed, confessing my panic that I wouldn't be able to do it properly.

Then I picked up the syringe, tapped the air bubbles to the top, squirted the air out, and tried again. And this time, it was successful!

During the two days that we were alone, Jess and I had the opportunity to talk sister-to-sister, going deeper than the surface-level topics we kept to when Mom and Jordan were around. We talked about her fears and anxiety, my life in Texas, and how much we had both changed. It felt good to just be us for a few moments. One afternoon, we sat on the balcony, listening to the waves and talking about the upcoming book tour.

"I'm not sure I should go on the book tour with Anna," I confessed, while watching the water crash onto the shore far below us. "I feel guilty going on a road trip while you're so sick. What if something happens and I can't get back?"

Jess stared out at the water from her chair beside me.

"Do you remember how we always wanted to take a road trip across the country?" she asked.

"Yes, we've talked about it forever," I answered.

"Go on the book tour," her voice was quiet but firm. "This is your chance to go cross-country. Go for me." I looked at her, tears in my eyes. She stared straight ahead.

"Okay," I whispered. "If you're sure, I will."

"Go," she told me again, turning her head to look at me.

I knew then that my travel-loving, wanderlusting sister had given me permission to continue living my life in a way that she could not live hers. She had always been the more adventurous of the two of us. Not only had she dragged me on dozens of random road trips and adventures, but she'd also backpacked multiple European countries on two different trips. Somewhere deep in our souls, we both knew the chances of us going on our cross-country road trip together were very slim. She gave me permission to go without her.

A few days later, we sat on the balcony again, this time discussing my wardrobe for the book tour. I needed Jess's fashion sense to help me overhaul my former teaching attire into something more suitable for a book tour manager.

"You need to go from tired teacher to savvy business woman," she advised.

Later the following week, Jess had a follow-up appointment at the Medical University of South Carolina. After the appointment, we drove back to SC, Mom and Jess in Mom's car and me alone in Jess's car. I spent much of the four-hour drive on the phone, processing my thoughts and emotions with a few close friends. I was scheduled to fly back to Texas on February 17. I spent my last few days in SC seeing friends and watching movies with Jess.

The day before I left, she had asked me to move a wingback armchair from the living room into her bedroom. Reclining at any angle was hard because her abdomen was so swollen that it was difficult for her to breathe if she wasn't sitting straight up. I moved the chair to her room, where she was curled up on her bed with her dog, a Shih Tzu-Maltese mix named Lola (Lola Chanel Montez, to be exact). A movie was quietly playing on her TV as she drifted in and out of sleep. I positioned the chair by her bed and sat down. We talked a little until she finally went to sleep. I sat in the chair for a while before I sneaked out of the room. I was meeting a friend for lunch that afternoon, and I knew Jess would sleep most of the day. We had planned to watch a movie together that night, but Jess was still groggy and sleepy from her pain meds. I poked my head in her door before I went to bed.

"Are you awake?" I asked

"Barely," she said from her bed.

"I just wanted to say goodnight and tell you bye since I'm leaving early in the morning," I said.

"You're leaving tomorrow? What day is it?" she replied.

"It's Thursday; tomorrow is Friday," I answered. "My flight leaves at 7:00 in the morning."

"Oh." Her voice sounded weighted and flat. The room was silent for a few seconds. I could tell she was struggling to stay awake.

"I love you, little buddy," I said. "I'll see you later."

"I love you, too," her voice whispered through the

darkened room. "Bye."

I backed up, pulling the door closed. As I stared at the door knob, the weight of leaving, of knowing that I might not see my sister again crashed into my chest, but I also knew I had to go. For me, and for her.

I flew back to Texas the next day with a heavy heart. Realistically, I knew my sister was very, very ill. But I was also trying to hold onto the last shreds of faith that a miracle was still possible. I wanted to hope even though the options seemed to be running out. Jess had finally decided to pursue surgery; the problem now, to my knowledge, was that there wasn't a surgeon who was willing to risk it since her body was so weak. But her options were limited, and time was running out.

Chapter 12:

The Epic Book Tour

Back in October 2016, Anna spoke at a conference in Tomball, Texas. Between sessions, we sat in the green room talking to another speaker, Charity, about Anna's upcoming book release. Anna mentioned that she was planning to go on a cross-country book tour.

"Who are you taking with you?" Charity asked.

"No one. I'm just going by myself," Anna replied.

Charity's eyes widened.

"You need someone to go with you! That's a lot of traveling to do alone."

I sat across the room, listening. Charity glanced over at me as I slowly raised my arm into the air.

"I volunteer as tribute," I offered as a solution.

Since early September, when Anna began seriously talking about going on a book tour, I had told myself I would go with her. I was already working as her assistant on a limited basis, mostly helping her edit her book, in addition to my part-time job as a behavioral therapist, and just assumed I would accompany her on the book tour the following summer.

"See!" Charity exclaimed. "You already have someone to go."

Anna looked at me, stunned.

"Really? I can't ask you to do that. You have a job."

"Yes, but not one that I'm overly attached to," I told her. "Let's talk about it."

Eventually — after months of conversations during which

Anna assured me she wouldn't dream of asking me to drop everything and go on the road for months and me assuring her that it was something I wanted to do — we agreed that I would accompany her on the road trip.

By the end of February 2017, we were busy planning Anna's book launch party and the first leg of the book tour. I spent the two weeks before the party finalizing details, organizing volunteers, coordinating lodging requests from out-of-town guests, and attempting to wrap my mind around an entire summer on the road. When the day of the launch party arrived, I was a bit frazzled, to say the least. After lunch with all the women from #the4500 who traveled to Dallas for the book launch, I led a group of volunteers to the Think Differently office where the party would take place that night. The team of volunteers worked together to quickly turn the office lobby into a space for book signing and mingling. When Anna walked in, we were thrilled to see the happiness on her face.

So many people showed up to celebrate her and her book that night. The building was packed with people, the crowd spilling out into the parking lot. And although I spent most of the night shaking from head to toe with all the adrenaline, being able to make sure the night went as smoothly as possible was a joy.

With the book's official release behind us, it was time to buckle down and map out the details of our road trip, both figuratively and literally. Armed with a list of names of people from #the4500 who had offered to host us, a list of bookstores that would prominently display *The Polygamist's Daughter*, and three previously-scheduled events in April, May, and June, I set out to plot a route around Texas, then west and north to Portland, east to New York and south back to Texas, then east to Pennsylvania and south to Florida, and all the stops in between.

We had a trial run on the first weekend in April when we packed up the car, drove to Temple where we stayed with our friend Taylor and her husband, then headed on to Austin for a book signing. A bunch of people we knew from #the4500, as well as Anna's friends and family came to celebrate with her. I was standing in the middle of the main aisle taking pictures of Anna at the book table and chatting with some friends from #the4500 when Jana, one of the #the4500mamas (a term of endearment bestowed upon the older and wiser members of the group) walked up behind me and said hello. Delighted to see her, I turned around to hug her. As she squeezed me, she whispered in my ear.

"I brought someone with me," she said mischievously, a twinkle glinting in her eye.

I pulled back, peering over her shoulder. Walking through the door behind her was Jen. *Jen Hatmaker was at Anna's book signing.* I gasped, my hand flying to my mouth as I spun around to look at Anna, who was facing the door.

When she looked up and saw who had arrived, her mouth dropped open. I lifted my camera from its place around my neck and started snapping as Jen approached the table, enveloped Anna in a tight hug, and then stepped back, laughing and smiling as Anna tried to recover from the shock of the moment. Anna had been in the middle of signing a book for someone, so Jen ran upstairs to sign her own books while Anna finished.

In the meantime, I ran out to the car to grab my advance reader copy (ARC) of Jen's new book, *Of Mess and Moxie*, that would be released later that summer. As Anna and I were pulling out of the driveway the day before, we'd realized neither of us had our ARCs and we were on a deadline to read them and submit our endorsements to the publisher. But Anna couldn't find hers, so we only had mine. I walked over to Jen, greeting her. Then I asked Jen if she would sign my ARC. She graciously agreed.

"Who should I sign it to?" she asked.

"Um, well, Anna will kill me if you don't sign it to both of us, so Anna and Ticcoa," I told her.

Laughing, she jotted a quick note, signed her name, and handed the book back to me. Later, when I opened it to see the inscriptions, I read:

To Anna and Ticcoa,

<3 you girls!

Jen Hatmaker

And that is the story of how Anna and I have shared custody of one of Jen Hatmaker's books!

We spent the night with one of Anna's sisters, then drove back home on Sunday, stopping for two quick coffee meetups with two different authors Anna followed on social media, Candice Curry and Chuck Tate. I also got a text from Mom that day, saying that Jess was headed back to the ER hoping to have another procedure to drain some of the fluid from her abdomen. When we arrived home, we had three days to finalize plans for the first half of the trip, which would last until early June when we needed to be back in Texas for two family events.

On Friday, April 7, we packed the SUV with books, clothes, air mattresses, and a variety of other essentials and hit the road again, this time starting in Houston before making our way west through and beyond Texas.

Our weekend in Houston began with a meet-and-greet at our #the4500 friend, Evelyn's, house on Friday. On

Saturday, we drove to the south side of Houston where Anna spoke at her literary agent's church: one of the most-attended gatherings on the tour.

On Sunday morning, we headed for that night's destination in Midland. On our way out of town, we stopped at one of the houses Anna lived in as a teenager and recreated a photo from her book. We also stopped at the Campbell Road house where Anna lived with her sister, Lillian, and brother-in-law, Mark, after she escaped her father's cult at thirteen.

When we arrived, Anna steered the SUV to a stop by the curb in front of the dilapidated house sitting clearly abandoned behind a chain link fence. A sign declared the building was to be destroyed soon. We climbed out of the car and peered past the fence. Anna posed by the mailbox and I took her picture. Slowly, we made our way down the sidewalk and around the corner. The chain link fence became a tall wooden fence. At the back side of the yard, the wooden gate stood slightly ajar. Anna looked at me.

"Should we go in?" she asked. "We should just go look at the yard."

I was skeptical, but curiosity won out. Anna slipped through the gate and I followed closely behind. I let her get a few steps ahead of me so I could take pictures as we walked across the yard toward the house. We kept our voices low, subconsciously trying to remain incognito.

When we reached the rear of the house, Anna peered through a couple of the windows, trying to identify the rooms from memory. She found the kitchen window and reminisced about the time she'd spent gazing out it as she washed dishes at the sink. The back door was a few steps to our right. It was slightly ajar. Anna turned to me again.

"Should we go in? she asked again. "It wouldn't be breaking and entering, just entering."

I was even more skeptical this time but also just as curious to see this piece of Anna's past. After weighing our options, we decided to take our chances with one caveat. We would tour the house on Facebook Live just in case anything happened. Anna handed me her phone and we went live, telling our friends where we were and what we were doing. Comments scrolled across the screen as some of them expressed excitement over our adventure and others told us to turn around and leave. I held the phone over Anna's head as she opened the door wider and stepped into the house.

The room we entered first was the office for the family's appliance business when Anna lived there with Mark and Lillian. She pointed out where his desk had sat and told me stories about how he ran the business. We made our way through the empty rooms, me recording while Anna reminisced. Eventually, we circled back to the office, but instead of heading outside, we stepped through the interior door to the garage. Debris and broken glass littered the floor, so we carefully picked our way to the laundry room attached to the garage. Inside the laundry room was a door leading to another small addition that had been Anna's room for a time when she lived in the house. Jokingly, Anna knocked on the door.

"Hello, is anyone there?" she called. "I'm going to open it," she said to me and the camera.

"Okay," I said nervously.

"I hope no one's in there," she mused. "Me, too!" I agreed.

The tension in the air was palpable as she turned the knob and pushed the door open. Her head blocked the camera as she peered through the doorway to see into the room.

"Oh!" she gasped, moving back toward me, allowing me to see into the room.

"Oh!" I echoed her surprise.

It was obvious someone was living in the room. There were a pair of boots sitting against the wall, a makeshift cardboard pallet bed in the middle of the floor, and a few other belongings that denoted someone's continuous presence in the room. I backed up, Anna closed the door, and we hurried back through the laundry room, garage, and office, and out the back door. Our friends watching the live video were commenting at a rapid pace, expressing their surprise, and telling us to get the heck out of there.

Walking at a brisk pace, we walked across the yard and squeezed through the gate. Once we were safely on the sidewalk again, we stopped to catch our breath. So far, this was the most adventurous thing we had done on the book tour. And it was only Day 9. Adrenaline pumping through our veins, we continued our drive out of Houston, stopped for quick meet-up in Katy with another #the4500 friend, and paused for a quick look at the Alamo and famed Riverwalk in San Antonio.

Monday, April 10, after stopping briefly in Lubbock, where our #the4500 friend Amanda met us in the parking lot of Barnes and Noble for a quick hug and to deliver a bag of road trip snacks, we crossed the state line into New Mexico, soon followed by Arizona. It was only Day 10 of the book tour, and already I was the farthest west I had ever been. We stayed in a hotel in Tucson that night, thanks to the generosity of one of our #the4500 friends. The next day, we drove to Casa Grande for a small event. On Wednesday, April 12, we spent the afternoon with our #the4500 friend Heidi. That night we arrived at Anna's brother's house where we were staying for a couple of nights. We were warmly welcomed and stayed up late playing cards with his family.

Early the next morning, I was awakened by my phone ringing. I rolled over in the twin bed in one of Anna's nieces' bedrooms. Eyes half-open, I fumbled for my phone and looked at the screen. It was Mom. I knew Jess had gone to the ER a few days before; the doctors had attempted to drain some of the fluid from her abdomen again. But the procedure had not gone well and the doctors had induced a coma to give her body some relief from the nonstop pain.

"Hello," I answered the phone.

"Hey," Mom said. "I wanted to let you know that Jess is not doing well. They've tried weaning the sedation drugs but she isn't waking up. We have to decide whether to take her off the ventilator."

Her words hit me like a ton of bricks. I felt like the wind had been knocked clean out of me.

"Okay, keep me posted," I said, knowing there was nothing I could do.

"I'm sorry I had to tell you this," Mom said. We hung up shortly and I climbed out of bed. Tears were starting to pool in my eyes. I walked down the hall to the room where Anna was staying. I knocked on the door and entered. Anna took one look at me and knew something was terribly wrong.

"What happened?" she asked, sitting up. I sat on the edge of the bed and relayed my conversation with Mom and the tears flooded out of my eyes. I bent forward and laid my head on the bed. Anna put her hand on my head as she sat there and cried with me. Then, she went into crisis management mode.

"I'll cancel my lunch plans today," she told me. "I can take you to the airport and put you on a plane to South Carolina."

"No, you don't have to cancel your plans," I replied. "And I don't think there's any reason for me to get on a plane immediately. There's nothing I can do to change the situation. This is where Jess would want me to be," I reasoned. "And she won't even know I'm there. If I left the book tour right now, she would beat me."

"Okay, but the minute you change your mind, I will put you on a plane," Anna promised. "That is always an option."

Anna went downstairs to get both of us coffee and let her brother and sister-in-law know briefly what was going on. Then she got dressed and ready for lunch while I drifted in and out of sleep. Mom called later that afternoon and asked if there was anything I wanted to tell Jess.

"Tell her I love her," I choked through my tears. "And that she has made me brave."

Chapter 13:

What Happened in Vegas

Later that evening, I dragged myself out of bed and went downstairs to have dinner with Anna and her brother's family, though I did not have much of an appetite. We played cards again that night, which helped distract me for a while. I will never forget the compassion and care Anna's brother and sister-in-law extended to me while we were in their home.

The next day, Friday, April 14, we set off for points north. We drove through Sedona, weaving our way through red rocks to the Grand Canyon. While we were on the road, my phone pinged frequently with updates from Mom; notifications from #the4500, who I had asked to pray; and phone calls from my closest friends offering to pay for plane tickets and do whatever I needed once I got to South Carolina. In the late afternoon, Anna and I arrived at the Grand Canyon. I stood at the edge, taking in as much of the view as I could, thinking to myself that I was experiencing it for both my sister and myself. We walked further down the path, away from the crowded overlook. I kept inching closer to the edge of the canyon.

"You're making me nervous," Anna said.

"It's fine, I'm not even that close to the edge," I told her, stepping off the path again. She jokingly grabbed at the sleeve of my cardigan.

"How am I going to explain your disappearance to your family if you fall off the edge of the cliff?" she asked.

"I may not be in the best state of mind, but I'm not going to fling myself into the Grand Canyon." I laughed. Then I climbed down onto a rock that stuck out over the chasm below and sat down with my feet at the edge to take a picture. Anna stood on safer ground above me.

As we turned to head to the gift shop, I spied a boulder

looming over the path on the non-canyon side. I climbed on top of it and instructed Anna to take my picture. I jumped down and looked at the picture. My arms were spread wide and the sun was directly behind me, so I was silhouetted in the picture. It's one of my favorite photos from the book tour because my pose and the rays of sun symbolize the elation I felt as seeing the Grand Canyon for the first time; the darkness that hides my face represents the sadness I felt.

Our destination for the night was Las Vegas. Anna and I had a mostly-unspoken understanding on the book tour: if we needed to get somewhere in a hurry or had to navigate big city traffic, she would drive. If she needed a break for a stretch of road that didn't involve those scenarios, I was happy to take the wheel. So, the fact that I was in the driver's seat as we approached Las Vegas was kind of a big deal for me. Neither of us had realized I'd be tasked with navigating Vegas traffic at night, and when we realized it, it was almost too late to do anything about it.

Anna did ask if I wanted to pull over and switch spots, but we were already in the thick of it and the thought of maneuvering to the shoulder made me more nervous than soldiering on. It was nerve-wracking, for sure, but I count weaving through the throngs of cars on a hundred-lane highway at night as one of my proudest accomplishments of the book tour. Those were tough days, y'all. Let me have the little things.

Groggily, I rolled over in the hotel bed and looked at my phone. 4:00 a.m. Two missed calls, three text messages, and a voicemail from Mom. Tears welled in my eyes and a knot formed in my stomach. "No, no, no," I whispered as my lungs constricted. I needed to call Mom back, but I already knew.

Trembling, I stumbled toward the bathroom. I grabbed a box of tissues and, fighting nausea, went back into the bedroom. *I have to wake her up. I can't do this alone.* I thought. Clutching my phone and tissue box in one hand, I carefully pulled back the blanket of the other bed.

"Anna," I whispered as I sat down. Startled, my friend opened her eyes. "Mom called. I don't want to call her back."

Tears pooled in her eyes.

She knew, too.

Anna put her arm around me as I pressed the button to return Mom's call.

"Jess passed away at 3:15 this morning," she told me.

I didn't hear anything else.

My little sister was gone.

Slipping away during the night, she'd taken the "second star to the right and straight on 'til morning," as J.M. Barrie wrote in *Peter Pan*, one of Jess's favorite books. In a hotel on the Las Vegas strip, my heart shattered into a million pieces that April morning.

When I hung up the phone, Anna held me close as I sobbed silently. My world was spinning out of control.

Around 9:30 Saturday night, we crossed the California state line. I whipped off my sleep mask just in time to see the blur of the sign as we drove by. I was exhausted in every way after such an early, emotionally-grueling start.

We arrived at our destination and were met warmly by Anna's sister, Sasha. Anna got out of the car first; this was normal since I took my time exiting and let her get all her squealing out of the way. I was a little longer than usual, though, and she poked her head back in and asked if I was getting out. I told her I'd be right behind her. She closed the door and followed Sasha into the house, informing her, I'm sure, on my current state. Slowly, I pulled the bags I would need for the night out of the car and went inside.

As I've struggled with anxiety over the last four-ish years, a weighted blanket has long been on my wish list. When I experience anxiety, I want nothing more than to burrow in bed under a heavy blanket. It's an innate need that calms me. And because I was still in such an unsettled emotional state, my anxiety was also heightened. All day, I'd wanted nothing more than to burrow, but that's hard to do in a moving vehicle.

Sasha hugged me as I entered the house and led me to the room where we'd be staying. One of the things I'm most grateful for looking back on those days is the fact that we stayed with so many of Anna's family members during the hardest part of the book tour. I was drowning in my grief, barely getting through each day while also juggling the logistics of getting back to SC for the memorial service and still managing the tour. But every one of Anna's siblings that we stayed with during those two weeks provided me with a soft place to land. They are all well-acquainted with grief and were so compassionate and generous, giving me as much space as I needed to mourn. I never felt like I had to mask my heartache in front of them.

The rest of the night is a blur, mostly because I went straight to bed. What I found was that the bed was equipped with a heavy down comforter that cocooned me just as I longed for all day.

The next morning, I awoke and was immediately hit by a tidal wave of grief. I also realized that it was Easter Sunday. Back then, the symbolism of that day juxtaposed with my sister's death was comforting in some ways. Now the connection is empty and feels unimportant. My faith and spiritual beliefs have morphed a great deal in the last two years.

I think this was the first time I really became aware of the gravity of my loss. After we left the hotel room in Vegas Saturday, Anna and I had kept ourselves busy and distracted as much as possible. But on Sunday, I woke up with an empty, unscheduled day ahead of me; I cried from the time I woke up that morning to the time I crawled back in bed.

Anna brought me coffee, then breakfast, and offered gentle words of understanding (not comfort, mind you — because what comfort would be adequate — but understanding). We talked about how this was the first time I'd lost someone close to me, and my first experience with grief.

We didn't have any solid plans that day and she encouraged — or, rather, insisted — that I stay in bed, rest, and write. She knew as well as I did that I needed to process some of the things swirling around my head.

I stayed put well into the afternoon until Anna came to check on me and see if I wanted to go out with her that evening. This was our chance to see Hollywood, including the infamous sign, so I said yes. I didn't bother putting on makeup, but I did throw on earrings. I shoved my sunglasses on my face to hide my swollen, leaking eyes and we set off.

We cruised down Sunset Boulevard, popped into Barnes and Noble to sign stock copies of Anna's book, and met up with Adam Hawk, a gamer Anna's sons knew. (She definitely got cool mom points for that meetup.) Adam served us yummy tacos and flan. Finally, we found the spot to take pictures of the Hollywood sign just before sunset. While we were standing on the side of the road awaiting our turn to take pictures, I glanced over my shoulder and saw a faint rainbow arched across the valley. The very sight of it was a balm for my languishing soul.

The next day, as we were preparing to leave, Sasha knocked on the open bathroom door where I was putting on my makeup.

"Hey," I said as she leaned against the door frame.

"I wanted to give you this," Sasha said. She held a green, metal container with a lid in her hands. Turning to face her, I saw faint tears glistening in her eyes.

"Don't let your memories of your sister get crushed," she told me. "Life will try to crush them, but don't let it. This box is to help them not get crushed, to protect them."

My own eyes were glistening when she handed the box to me.

"Thank you," I whispered, the unspoken words between us acknowledging the shared experience of losing someone we loved.

Quietly, Sasha turned and slipped out of the room. I looked at myself in the mirror, realizing that wearing makeup was probably not a wise choice for the foreseeable future. Later, when Anna and I were packing our belongings back into the car, she saw the box.

"What's that?" she inquired.

"A gift from Sasha," I replied. "I'll tell you about it later."

My words stuck in my throat, thick with the gravity of the moment Sasha and I had together. It was a sacred moment, one that still brings tears to my eyes.

We made our way up the coast, stopping at Pismo Beach to dip our toes in the Pacific Ocean. Our next stop was Monterey, where we spent the night with our Twitter friend Rebecca. Tuesday morning, we were scheduled to stay with her parents in the San Francisco area. That evening, we had a small event at our friend Janine's home.

During our event, I checked my phone and saw a missed call and text from Mom asking me to call her as soon as possible. Excusing myself from the group, I walked to the guest bedroom. I called Mom back and she relayed her current frustration with convincing my father to sign the release form for my sister's remains to be cremated. Once again, I was thrust into the middle of their disagreements. Jess had never hidden her wishes to be cremated; she'd talked openly about it since she was a teenager. I hung up the phone and texted him, saying that he was doing far more harm than good to any fragments of relationship he had with his other children and that he should just sign the $#%& paper. Without waiting for a response, I put my phone on silent again, took a few deep breaths, and left the guest room.

I was so angry at being thrust into the middle of their argument but I also needed to put that aside for the next few hours in order to do my job. Just before I left the guest room, Anna came in to grab something and I quickly told her what was going on. Simply being able to voice my frustration helped release some of my anger for the moment.

The next morning, we had some downtime and I had a weighty task to complete: writing my sister's obituary. After talking about the difficulty of the situation, Anna sat with me while I opened my laptop and stared at a blank screen

"I can't do this," I whispered. We sat in silence for a few minutes. Finally, Anna offered help in a way that mirrored my own when I'd watched her struggle with the final edits for her book the previous fall.

"Hand me your laptop," she said, reaching for it. "You tell me what to write and I'll type it."

I relinquished the laptop, curled my hands around my coffee cup, and began telling her what I wanted to say.

We spent the next day sightseeing in San Francisco with Janine. She took us to the Golden Gate Bridge, Fisherman's Wharf, Lombard Street, and Facebook headquarters in Menlo Park, where Anna tried to talk the security guard into letting us see inside the building. We had a blast. Still, I cried all day, keeping my red, swollen eyes hidden behind my sunglasses. I never heard anything from my father, but Mom texted a couple of days later that he had signed the release form.

On Thursday, April 20, we left San Francisco. Our original plan was to drive through the redwood forest and spend the night in Eureka, but we woke up that morning to news that mudslides had made our route inaccessible. So, we decided to drive straight to our next destination, Anna's sister's house in Portland, a day ahead of schedule.

For the next three days, I was a hermit, keeping mostly to myself in the room where we were staying. This was the first long stretch of downtime we had since Jess died, and I collapsed. I cried, I slept, I stared into space. Anna brought me coffee, food, and wine as needed, and encouraged me to rest.

On our third day there, Anna asked if I wanted to go to dinner with her, her sister, and her brother-in-law, and I felt ready to emerge from my grief cave for a few hours. Even though sadness permeated my whole being, I enjoyed our meal together.

The next day, Kathleen and Jim took us to Cannon Beach. During the drive, I fell in love with the Oregon landscape — winding roads, lush green trees. It was overcast and cold that day, with a layer of fog shrouding the rocks along the beach that gave the coastline a subdued aesthetic. Bundled in my hoodie, I cradled my camera in my hands and searched for hidden detail through the lens, as I had learned from Jess. She was a talented photographer with a creative eye, always on the lookout for unique angles and perspectives. As I captured crabs scurrying across the beach, seagulls prancing along the wet sand, waves rolling onto shore, and silhouettes of majestic rocks rising from the water, I felt the nearness of her essence. Leaving the beach that day, I felt calmer.

On Monday, April 24, Anna had a joint podcast interview with her cousin, Ruth Wariner. To say I was excited to meet Ruth in person, after we'd helped launch her book, is a gross understatement. The following night, a local bookstore held a joint book signing and Q&A with Anna and Ruth. Watching these two cousins sharing their stories side-by-side was particularly moving. Both of them had overcome so many obstacles in their lives to be sitting in that bookstore together. The store was packed that night. A handful of friends from #the4500 were among the attendees and we all went out to celebrate with Ruth, her husband, Anna's sister, and brother-in-law after the signing.

The next morning, tired but energized by the excitement of the previous night, we left Portland en route to Twin Falls, Idaho for a quick overnight stay and a book signing at Barnes and Noble that our friend, Paige, arranged. Then we were off to Salt Lake City, where Anna and I would part ways for a few days. I was headed back to South Carolina for my sister's memorial service and she would continue the book tour in Utah.

As we drove to SLC that morning, Anna spoke encouraging words to me, reminding me that I had everything I needed to get me through the next few days. We pulled up to the terminal, and I grabbed my suitcase out of the truck. Anna met me at the back of the car where we snapped a quick selfie. She hugged me tight and we both had tears in our eyes when we parted. I turned and walked into the airport, dreading the trip ahead. During the flights from SLC to Dallas and Dallas to Greenville, I wrote the eulogy I would give at the service. I arrived in Greenville late Thursday evening, exhausted.

The memorial service was scheduled for Saturday morning at our former church, the one pastored by Pastor C. His daughter, Amber, who was also the worship leader, was coming to Mom's house Friday morning to finalize plans for the service. I sat at the kitchen table with them for a while before leaving to shop for something to wear to the memorial service. Basic black was *not* an option for a service in memory of my uniquely stylish sister.

I woke up in my sister's room early Saturday morning, already tired. Two of my #the4500 friends were driving to Greenville from Georgia and North Carolina to support me and represent the group in person. We were meeting for a quick breakfast before the service. Channeling Jess, I did my hair and makeup; then I put on the hot pink leggings I'd bought the day before, topped by the black tunic I'd brought with me. I finished my outfit with a floral kimono, silver wire feather earrings, and a matching necklace I swiped from Jess' closet, half-afraid she might send a lightning bolt to strike me for going through her stuff.

Grabbing the keys, my purse, and the printed eulogy, I got into Jess's car. I turned the radio on and headed to meet Camille and Candice. After a quick breakfast of chicken biscuits, they followed me to the church.

A few church members who were helping set up stopped to hug me and offer their condolences in the hallway as I led my friends to the sanctuary, which was decorated with flowers, balloons, and several huge framed pictures of Jess. An eclectic mix of music from her playlists — including Elvis, Hanson, *NSYNC, classic rock, pop, indie, etc. — was playing as well. (Jess's musical taste ran wide.) The pictures stopped me in my tracks. I let myself stare at them for a moment before I turned back to Camille and Candice. Amber approached and told me the rest of the family was waiting in the nursery. I followed her down the hallway to the room. I opened the door and walked into the room.

My family, sitting in folding chairs that lined three of the walls, greeted me. Then Amber gave us a quick rundown of the order of the service and said she would be back in a few minutes to usher us into the sanctuary. When she returned, there was a moment of awkwardness as no one stepped forward to line up first. My aunt looked at me.

"Lead the way, Ticcoa," she said.

So, I did. I led my family into the packed, dimly-lit sanctuary, walking past rows and rows of people who came to remember my sister's short life. We walked to the front center rows of the sanctuary and sat. I was seated on the far left, my brother, Josh, seated to my right. Several large pictures of Jess sat directly in front of me. Throughout the service, I alternated staring into her dark, familiar eyes and avoiding them entirely.

During the more difficult parts of the service, including Pastor Thomas's welcome, I found myself gripping Josh's leg, willing myself to breathe. Public speaking is something I do not enjoy at all, but I managed to stand before the crowd and speak twice during the service. The first time, occurring early in the service, was to read the tribute Anna had written to Jess, summarizing meeting Jess, becoming the president of her fan club, and her quest to gain Jess as a Twitter follower. The second time came after a slideshow of pictures that included many of the adventures we shared. This time, I was giving a eulogy.

Writing the eulogy was the second hardest thing I had ever written, after her obituary. But I felt proud of myself, and knew that she would've been proud of me, too, as I shared my memories with those who were gathered to remember her.

After the service, I went back to Mom's to take a nap and change clothes, then left to meet Dr. Drummond for an early dinner. We sat and talked while I booked my return flight to Salt Lake City for the following afternoon.

When I left the book tour, I'd booked a one-way flight, giving myself the option of staying in South Carolina up to a week, meeting back up with Anna in Denver. But after the memorial service, I felt like I needed to get back on the road for a variety of reasons. The most compelling reason was that Jess had encouraged me to go on this trip in the first place. And because we had wanted to take a cross-country road trip, I felt I was honoring her memory and spirit by continuing my travels. I needed to see the country for both of us. Plus, I also had her road trip mascot, Migrating Monty, in my possession now. He was the first possession of Jess's that I requested after she died. I'd texted Mom a few days before I arrived in South Carolina and asked her to find him so I could bring him back with me for the rest of the book tour. Another reason I wanted to get back on the road was that our next stop was Hildale/Colorado City, an infamous fundamentalist Mormon town on the border of Arizona and Utah. Anna had been invited to speak at the public library there, and it was such a momentous stop that I knew I would regret missing that part of the tour. So, I booked my flight back to Utah for Sunday night. It was time to get back on the road and make Jess proud.

Chapter 14:

The Worst/Best Summer of Endless Miles

On Sunday morning, I got up early and met Christine, for breakfast. We sat at Panera Bread Co. and talked for several hours, catching up on each other's lives. Then I headed back to Mom's to finish packing before catching my flight. My flight back to Salt Lake City is a blur in a memory. I was exhausted and drifted in and out of sleep, disoriented by hopping several time zones, and slightly unnerved by the worst turbulence I'd experienced. I arrived in Utah and met up with Anna around midnight. On Monday morning, May 1, we left Anna's sister's house and drove south to the Hildale Public Library. As soon as we got in the car, I put Monty on the dashboard, where he spent the next three months as we crisscrossed the country.

We arrived at the small, white building in the early afternoon and went in to meet the library manager. She showed us the room where Anna would speak. While she and Anna chatted about the event, I set up the book table. Anna had enlisted the help of her social media followers to donate books to those who attended the gathering in Hildale. Forty books were covered within twenty-four hours. A few minutes after the appointed start time, two women, dressed in long, plain dresses entered the room. I sat at the table by the door and offered each of them a book, letting them know that we were giving them to attendees. Anna came over to greet them and introduce herself, then they seated themselves in the second row of folding chairs. More people trickled in, including a distant relative of Anna's who was not part of the fundamentalist community but also lived in Hildale.

As Anna began to answer questions from the women there, a few of them took out their cell phones and texted friends, telling them to come to the library. Slowly, more women showed up. Not all of them stayed the entire time, but we gave away thirty-five books during the event. Anna left the remaining books with her relative to give away. Watching Anna interact with the women of Hildale and leave her book with many of them was a definite highlight of the whole book tour — one I am glad I witnessed.

The next three months were both really hard and very exciting. We met so many #the4500 sisters for the first time and reunited with many more we had already met in person. I met Anna's mom and many more of her siblings, which was another highlight of the trip. Anna's third-grade teacher came to her Denver book signing. We sampled dozens of varieties of torte in Wisconsin and ate deep dish pizza and Chicago-style hot dogs. We visited Anna's publishing team at Tyndale. We had events in Colorado, Nebraska, Minnesota, Iowa, Wisconsin, and Indiana. We took longer breaks to rest in family and friends' homes in New York, Ohio, and Pennsylvania. An unexpected lull in plans gave us several days in Boston, so I dragged Anna to my favorite literary sites in Concord, MA. Alcott, Emerson, Thoreau, and Hawthorne, oh my!

In mid-May, we visited our friend, Xamayta, in Pennsylvania. While there, we attended her book club. They had read Anna's book and were eager to meet and discuss it with her. We were sitting around the table in the hostess' home when Xamayta cocked her head to the side and looked at me.

"Where did you get that?" she asked, gesturing to the bracelet encircling my wrist. My chin was resting in my palm. I lifted my head and touched the bracelet.

"It was my sister's," I replied. "I found it in her stuff when I was home for the memorial service." Xamayta's eyes widened.

"I sent it to her months ago," she said. "I saw it in a store and thought of her."

Tears sprang to my eyes as she spoke. The other women at the table had grown quiet, realizing Xamayta and I were having a moment. Knowing my sister had been loved and cared for by people who only knew her through me was endearing.

After leaving Pennsylvania we drove back to upstate New York to tour Niagara Falls and attend Anna's sister's graduation from Cornell. We spent a few days with some of Anna's siblings, then raced back to Texas for Anna's youngest daughter's graduation, her oldest daughter's wedding, and several media appearances.

Two weeks later, on June 15, we were back on the road for Leg 2. Our first stop was in Louisiana, followed by

Tennessee. Next, we went to my hometown of Greenville, SC, where I got to introduce Anna to my family and friends. We did several events there and Anna experienced a Southern, home-cooked Sunday dinner at my grandparents' house. We went north for events in Virginia and Maryland before returning to Pennsylvania, where we spent the Fourth of July. Traveling south again, we spent one night in Columbia, SC for a book club at our friend Catherine's house before continuing to Florida. We watched a sunrise on the beach with our friend, Beverly, met one of Anna's distant cousins, and spent an afternoon by ourselves on a private Gulf Coast beach. Then we spent a few days in Georgia for an event and time with more #the4500 friends before heading home to Texas for a few days of rest and an event at a local church.

For our final leg of the book tour, we arrived in Oklahoma on July 21, had an event the next day, and left for New Mexico on my birthday, July 23. We stopped for lunch with Anna's friend and mentor, Carolyn (who had been our roommate at Splendid in the Hills), at the infamous Big Texan restaurant in Amarillo. We spent the night in Albuquerque on our way back to Salt Lake City for our last event on the book tour.

Once there, we spent four days attending the Sunstone Symposium where Anna spoke. I then spent three days in New Mexico at my friend Kelli's house while Anna made a solo trip to her birthplace in Mexico. When she returned to the States, we reunited in El Paso and headed home to Texas one more time after the 112 days; 23,461 miles; 40 states; and two countries that comprised the #EpicBookTourTPD over four months.

While I needed the busyness of the book tour to keep me from spiraling into a dark hole that I feared I would never crawl out of, I was also an introvert who was sleeping in a different place every two to three nights, putting on a brave smile for events several times a week, and coordinating upcoming events from the passenger seat. I had a job to do and that was my saving grace. But to say it was simple would be grossly inaccurate. I wore sunglasses constantly for weeks, hiding swollen eyes. For weeks after I rejoined the book tour, I spent much of our drive time sleeping as Anna drove. It was exhausting.

Looking back on that time now, I can see how it mirrored my experience after the Gallaudet incident. I was grieving deeply, I was depressed, my anxiety was high, and I was pushing through as best I could. I wasn't in denial that my sister had died, but I did realize that I needed something to do. Had I been in South Carolina that summer or home alone in Texas while Anna was on the book tour alone, I would have collapsed. I truly doubt I would have made it out of that grief alive. Just as #the4500 had saved me two years before, the book tour had saved me this time.

I hadn't felt pressured, by Anna or anyone else, to get

back on the road and continue the book tour before I was ready. I knew I would regret not finishing the book tour. I wanted to commemorate the brave life Jess had led, to memorialize her adventurous spirit that had spilled over into my soul, and to represent her memory well. I couldn't imagine a better way to honor her life than by embracing my own adventurous spirit and continuing to live my life as best I could given the circumstances. And I believe I did just that with the help of Anna, my friends, the sisterhood of #the4500, and the book tour.

It was both the worst and the best summer of endless miles.

Epilogue

"Do *not* get tattoos in Vegas!" I heard our friend Jana implore Anna through the speakerphone.

A year earlier, when my siblings ganged up on me and tried to convince me to get a tattoo with them, I dug in my heels and refused, firm in my no tattoos on my body stance. Suddenly, though, there was no question in my mind. I was getting a tattoo to memorialize my sister.

At first, I considered a shooting star because Jess had been talking about getting a star tattoo for months and now, I thought of her as a shooting star streaking across the sky. But I've never actually liked the shape of stars. So, there I was, sitting in the main room of our Las Vegas hotel room, browsing the internet for said tattoo shops. Just hour earlier, we'd awoken to the news that Jess was gone. As the new reality of living in a world without my sister settled over me, the desire to absorb the essence of who she is and was flooded every fiber of me. I couldn't let her go. I couldn't let her be forgotten. I couldn't let her slip away completely. From the other room, I heard Jana speaking in her authoritative professor voice.

"I'll make an appointment with my guy. You can get them while you're here in Minnesota, if you still want them, and you'll have time to think about what you really want," she continued.

"Okay, fine. We won't get tattoos today," Anna agreed.

Two weeks later, we arrived in the small town where Jana lived. Our tattoo appointment was booked for the following day, May 11, 2017: Day 41 of the Epic Book Tour. Jana took us to her favorite coffee shop and then we headed to the tattoo parlor. She introduced us to the tattoo artist, Kevin. I had emailed pictures of what I wanted, so he asked me questions about size and placement. When he came back from the printer with a copy of the image that was about three inches tall, I laughed.

"Um, I'm gonna need that to be smaller," I said, gesturing on my wrist to a space slightly larger than the size of my thumbnail.

"Oh, so you want it to be barely visible?" he quipped.

"Exactly!" I shot back.

He went back to the computer and returned with a printout of the image that closer matched the size I had envisioned.

"Perfect!" I declared when he placed it on my wrist.

While he and I were negotiating the size of my tattoo, Anna and Jana were browsing the binders full of designs. Anna had not fully decided on what tattoo she wanted.

"I don't want to have to look at it every day," she told us. "I want it somewhere that I can't see it all the time."

After asking Kevin a few questions about location, she decided on a small red heart outlined in black for her ankle. It was the perfect choice for her, since she always draws a small heart by her name when she signs copies of her book for her readers. Decisions made, the three of us followed Kevin into the back room, the two of us who had always been opposed to tattoos now ready to etch these meaningful symbols into our skin.

Anna sat next to me as Kevin cleaned my wrist and began inking the design into my skin. It hurt, but not terribly, and it only took two minutes to complete. Jana stood behind us and snapped a couple of pictures. Kevin wiped away the excess ink and Anna took a picture of my wrist before he wrapped the tattoo.

Next, Anna hopped onto the table and twisted so that her ankle was facing up. She grimaced as Kevin began tattooing the heart on the fleshy spot behind her ankle bone while I captured the whole process on Facebook Live, per Anna's wishes. Jana moved around behind me, taking pictures and cracking jokes.

After Anna's tattoo was finished, we left the shop and went to lunch. All afternoon and evening, I kept staring at my wrist, permanently etched with a reminder of my sassy sister: a logo she had created for herself years ago from her initials, in her loopy, cursive handwriting.

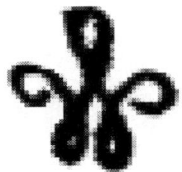

It wasn't until we were in Ohio the following week that I realized what the tattoo resembled.

Her initials — JL — created a five-point shape.

A star.

Jess is my forever star, a guiding spark in my life.

And just as I carried her with me throughout the

remainder of the worst and best summer of endless miles, I will carry her memory for the rest of my life. My brothers, Josh and Jordan, whose first and last initials are also JL, are with me, too. The four of us are entwined together, even as I live my life unbound.

Afterword

Dear Friend,

Thank you for reading this book. The process of writing and publishing *Unbound* took longer than I expected, but it was birthed when both I and it were ready. It is a book whose story I have held closely to my heart. Now, it is alive in the world for all to read. Already, I have watched as the story of freedom, friendship, grief, sorrow, and sisterhood you just read gives others permission to live their lives, fully and without apology. I hope my experiences speak deeply to you, as well.

Life is often messy, disjointed, and untidy. If you found any part of this story to be so, know that it felt that way because that is what I experienced as I lived through these events. Though we desperately ache for a pretty bow to tidy the loose ends of our stories, that's not always possible. Our lives, our stories, are still full of beauty: places where the light shines through our cracks. This story is one of the brightest lights in my life. It reminds me where I once was, who I used to be, and how much my life has changed — geographically, mentally, relationally, emotionally, and spiritually. My former self was as strong and brave as she knew how to be and I am so proud of her for never giving up, even when she couldn't see her way back to the light.

Those of you who have met me in real life or engaged with me online may wonder about the events that have occurred in the three years between the end of this book and its publication. Perhaps you hoped to read about my spiritual deconstruction and reconstruction within these pages. But I felt strongly that this was not the book to address those things. My approach to spirituality and faith has changed much, but I did not want that topic to distract from the sacredness of this book. I began writing *Unbound* in 2016 and finished in 2020. I am not the same person today that I was when I began this book. But I still believe wholeheartedly in its importance and the validity of its message.

Unbound: A Story of Freedom and Sisterhood is an undeniable mile marker in my life. It is a call for others to embrace their lives and honor their deepest desires. My hope is that you walk away from this book with courage to break the ties that bind you to the expectations others have for you, determination to reclaim what has been robbed from you, and permission to confidently live your own life. Even when it is hard, even when the circumstances and timing make little sense to anyone else. May you be unbound.

Ticcoa

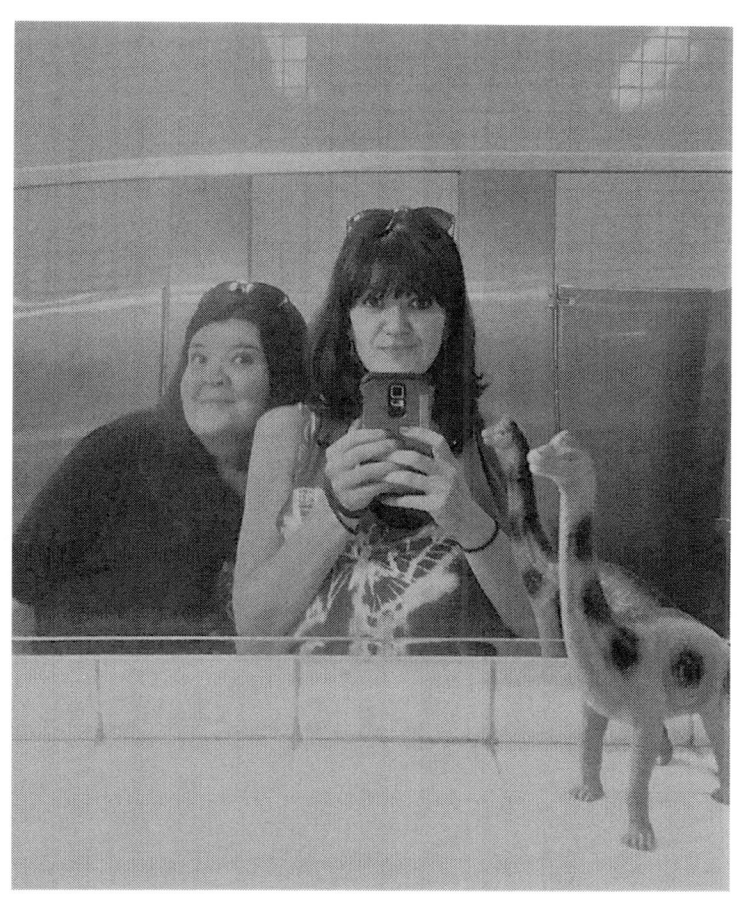

Ticcoa, Jess, and Monty en route to Texas

June 2016

Courtesy of Jessica Leister

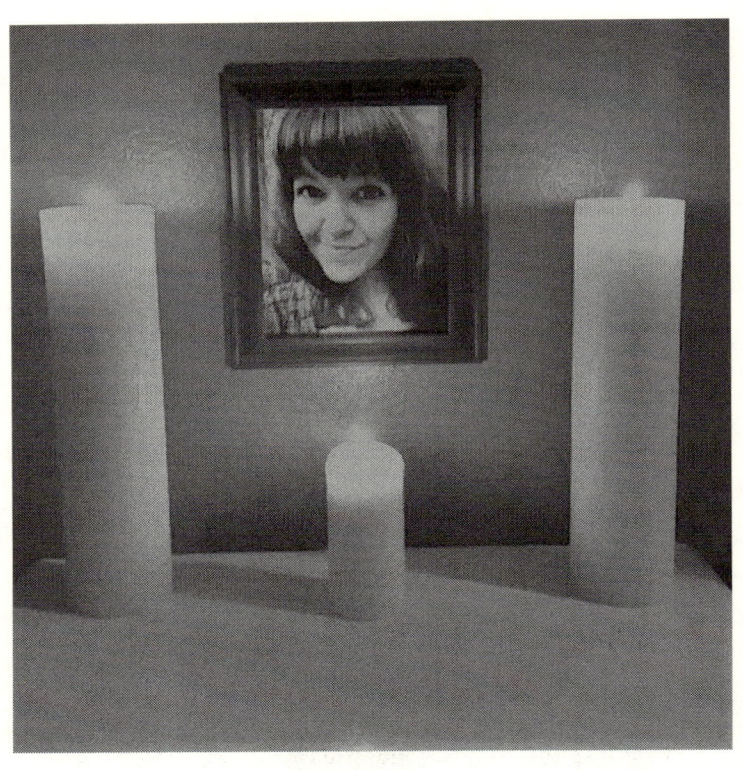

Jess, forever enshrined in our hearts. This is the autographed picture she sent Anna, aka "her biggest fan" in April 2016.

Courtesy of Jessica Leister

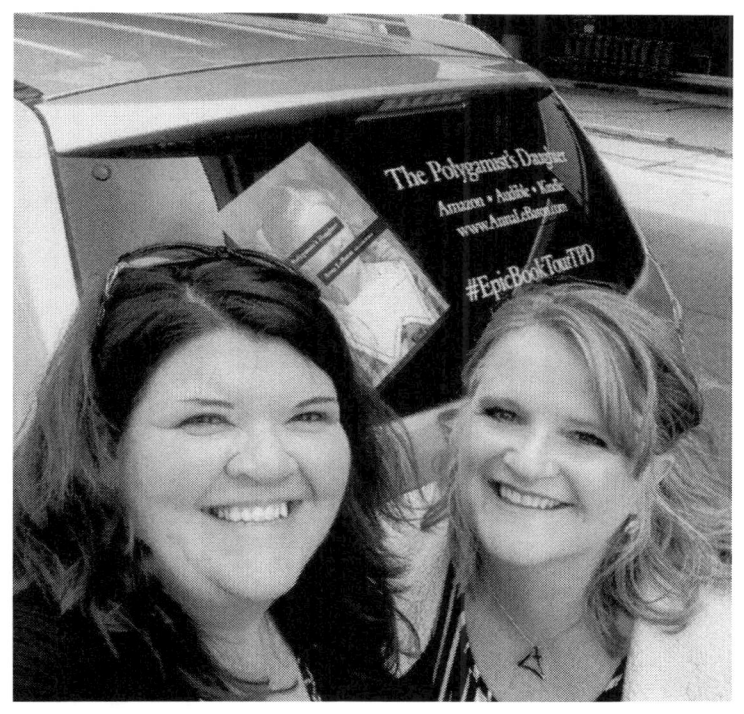

Ticcoa and Anna on the #EpicBookTourTPD, Salt Lake City airport, April 2017. I was on my way to South Carolina for Jess's memorial service.

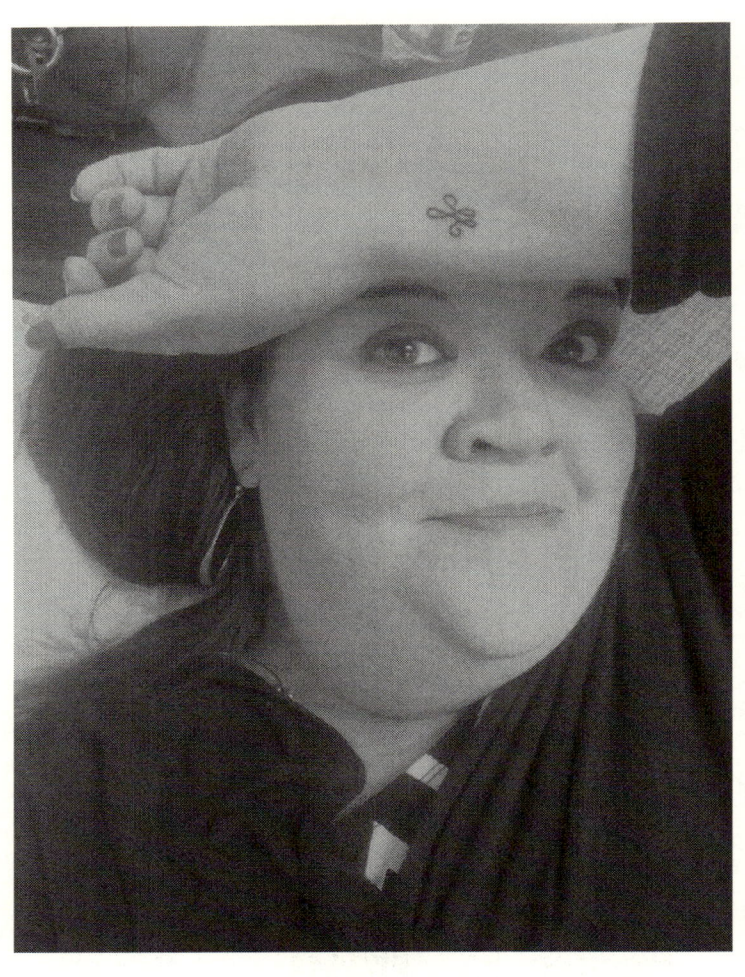

*Me and my newly-inked tattoo of Jess's
initials, Wisconsin, May 2017.*

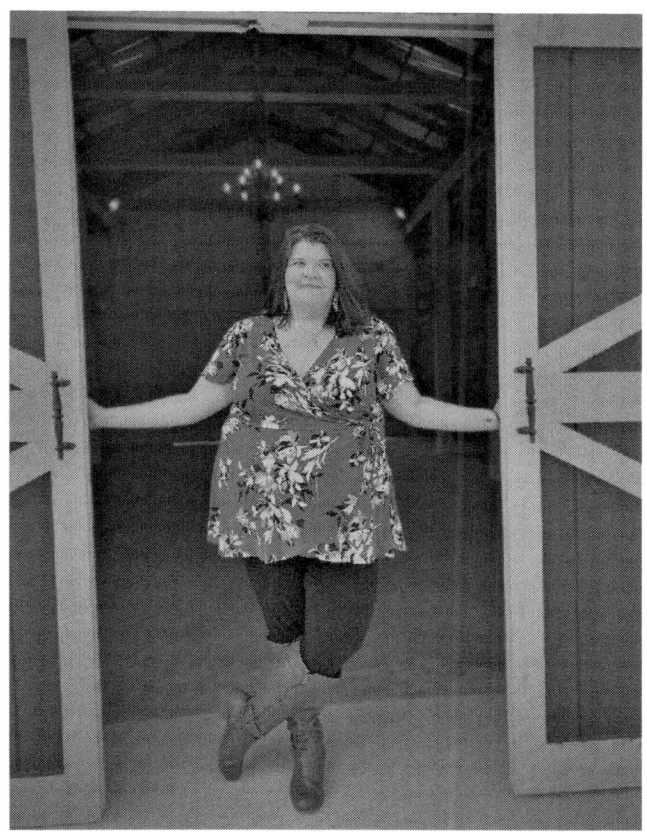

This photo, and the one on the front cover, symbolizes the freedom I've found in living an unbound life. VFF Retreat, Texas, December 2019.

Courtesy of Stephanie Dove Blake

Acknowledgments

There are so many people who have aided my journey to publication. If I tried to name you all, these acknowledgments would go on forever. But there are some whose support bears shouting from the rooftops. My gratitude knows no bounds (I suppose you could say it is unbound) for:

Bethany Beams, who hit the pavement running when I finally got my act together and formatted and edited this book. Trusting you with my book baby was easy because I knew you would make it the best it could be.

Nicole Grimes, who took my vision for the book cover and created a design beyond what I could imagine. Who knew TikTok would lead to such a treasure? It's just beyond appropriate that you designed both Anna's book cover and mine.

Ruth Spzunar, Goodreads guru, who took one more thing off my to-do list. Librarians rock!

My Patrons of the Literary Arts, wow! Your generosity and good faith in this project has astounded me. I couldn't have pulled this off so quickly without your support.

The Core Four, who helped me sharpen my writing skills, taught me to think critically, encouraged me to follow my heart, and became the best professors-turned-friends:

Dr. Julia Drummond, for taking this freshman wallflower under your wing and shepherding me through my college career as an advisor, teacher, mentor, and friend. And most importantly, for believing in my desire to bring ASL to NGU. You have my whole heart forever.

Dr. Catherine Sepko, for saying yes to my and Dr's D's idea to write an ASL course proposal. Our first meeting intimidated me; little did I know, I had entered a friendship with one of the wisest women I know. Your faith in me has kept me going on countless occasions. Our chats on the White Hall porch will forever be among my most treasured memories.

Dr. Becky Thompson, for the hundreds (thousands?) of notes you scrawled in colorful ink across the pages of my assignments, your generous spirit, compassionate ear, wise advice, and deep friendship. The hours spent in both your classroom and office were invaluable to becoming who I am today. Clear a chair for me, soon, okay?

Dr. Cheryl Collier, for saying yes to my independent study and giving me the opportunity to go rogue and write a course proposal as an undergraduate student. Your blunt truth-bombs scared me for a long time, but I am ever grateful for your leadership and friendship. Also, thanks for teaching me that every story doesn't need a pretty bow. It's still really difficult to leave them untied.

Christine Gaynor, for welcoming me into your classroom and being one of the best friends I have ever had. I know you don't like public accolades, but there was no way I was leaving you out. I'll just say this: I have zero regrets about working with you for six years. We really were a dynamic duo.

Asa, Henry, and every one of my students who passed through the doors of A3. You taught me so much about living life outside the box, without regard to other people's expectations. I am a better person because you were part of my life. And tell your parents Ms. Ticcoa says thanks for sharing you with her.

My family, especially Mom, Josh, Jordan, Grandma, Grandpa, Uncle Steve, Aunt Trina, Kasey, Eric, Olgui, Sofia, and Emma, for wholeheartedly supporting my move to Texas, even when it was brutally hard to say, "see you later." I love you all so much. Ohana.

My VFFs: Anna, Madlin, Stephanie, Celia, Jenny, Melissa, and Lauren: This book is finally done because of our goal-setting retreats. I came into your circle four years ago with no idea how to set and achieve big, hairy, audacious goals. Look at me, now! It took a while, but I think I'm getting the hang of this.

The Heyen kids: David, Caleb, Jacob, Kristina, and Hannah, who have wholeheartedly welcomed their mom's internet friend into their family. You all know who is my favorite kid. ;)

The LeBaron siblings who took such good care of me during the book tour. Your tenderness, compassion, and empathy touched the deepest places of my heart. You have all suffered much but are also the strongest, most generous people I have ever met.

Bob Hamp, for your commitment to teaching biblical truth in new ways and inviting people to think, live, lead, and learn differently. I'm so grateful for the role you have played in my journey to becoming unbound.

Jen Hatmaker (and her publishing team), for saying no to a 5,000-person launch team. It was the most providential no of my life. Being on the "B team" flipped my life upside down in the best possible ways. I have learned so much from you about fiercely standing up for what you believe and living with unapologetic. Plus, I found my circle of elephants because of you and #the4500. I am forever grateful.

#the4500. Wow. I will never, ever have enough words to express how much I love you girls. You busted into my quiet, boring little life and made yourselves at home--and I couldn't be happier that you did. You're my favorite internet friends, the pack of sisters I never expected. You circled up when I needed you most, and my life would not be the same without you. #the4500forLYFE

Tracy Page, the best hashtag-thief in all the land, for creating a safe, silly, spirited room for us to gather. And for using your gifts to create in-person retreats that allowed us to hug each other's' necks, look into each other's eyes, share our stories face-to-face, and deepen these unlikely friendships.

Anna LeBaron... I'm already choked up. "Thank you" doesn't begin to cover the vastness of my gratitude to and for you. The light radiating from you was so bright even in my dream that it pushed back the darkness and helped me find my way back to the path. This book is a testament to the miracle of our friendship; my story would be so different without you. You've played many roles in my life, but one of my favorites is Book Doula. You have held my hand throughout this process, offering both gentle and stern encouragement, reminding me to breathe when I am overwhelmed, and sitting with me in the pain that comes from transferring one's heart to the page. This book would not exist without your help birthing it. You are the sister I didn't know I needed, and you showed up exactly when I needed you most. I'm so glad you didn't just stay over there in your corner of the internet. I love you with my whole heart.

And, finally, for Jess, my first and best sister. I miss you every minute of the day. I am so grateful for the life we shared and the memories I hold of our adventures together. The hole you left in my life will never be filled. Thank you for releasing me to Texas with conviction and the instruction to fully embrace my life, and for hand-delivering me to my new home. It means the world to me. If you thought I'd been abducted by aliens back in 2016, you would be flabbergasted now! I love you forever, Little Buddy. (P.S. I threw an "Easter egg" into this book just for you! I think it would make you proud.)

Notes

Prologue

1. Habakkuk 2:2 NIV

2. 1 Corinthians 3:6-7 ESV

Chapter 3

1. Brown, Brene. Daring Greatly: How the Courage to Be Vulnerable Transforms the Way We Live, Love, Parent, and Lead. New York: Avery-Penguin Random House, 2012. p. 1

2. ibid. p. 58

3. ibid.

Chapter 5

1. John 11:38-44 NKJV

2. Hamp, Bob. Think Differently, Lead Differently: Bringing Reformation in Your Heart, Your Home and Your Organization. Thinking Differently Press, 2014. p. 40

3. Hamp, Bob. "A Kingdom Parable." Apple Podcasts. (No longer available.)

Chapter 6

1. Brown, Brene. Daring Greatly: How the Courage to Be Vulnerable Transforms the Way We Live, Love, Parent, and Lead. New York: Avery-Penguin Random House, 2012. p. 117

About the Author

A Carolina girl transplanted to Texas, Ticcoa Leister is an introvert who survived her Worst/Best Year on a 23,461-mile road trip with an extrovert. She's a literary nerd who has a weakness for 19th-century American authors, large bodies of water, cheesecake, Harry Potter, feather earrings, and a good cocktail. Ticcoa has learned to courageously embrace her life and loves sharing her story in hope that it will inspire others.

Find Ticcoa Online:
Facebook/Instagram/Twitter
@ticcoaleister
www.ticcoa.com

Find Migrating Monty Online:
Instagram
@migrating_monty

Made in the USA
Middletown, DE
08 November 2020

23573221R00120